AIDS

PERSONAL STORIES IN PASTORAL PERSPECTIVE

*Earl E. Shelp, Ronald H. Sunderland &
Peter W.A. Mansell, M.D.*

The Pilgrim Press
New York

Unless otherwise indicated, the biblical quotations in this book are from the *Revised Standard Version of the Bible*, copyright 1946, 1952, and © 1971, 1973 by the Division of Christian Education, National Council of Churches, and are used by permission. The quotation marked NEB is from *The New English Bible*, © The Delegates of the Oxford University Press and the Syndics of the Cambridge University Press, 1961, 1970, and is used by permission. Words of "Wind Beneath My Wings" are © 1982 Bobby Goldsboro Music Inc. and House of Gold Music Inc. and are used by permission of Warner Bros. Music. All rights reserved.

Library of Congress Cataloging-in-Publication Data

AIDS, personal stories in pastoral perspective.

Bibliography: p. 201.
1. AIDS (Disease)—Religious aspects.   2. AIDS (Disease)—Case studies.   3. Pastoral medicine.
I. Shelp, Earl E., 1947–   .   II. Sunderland, Ronald, 1929–   .   III. Mansell, Peter W. A.
[DNLM: 1. Acquired Immunodeficiency Syndrome—personal narratives.   2. Acquired Immunodeficiency Syndrome—psychology—personal narratives.   WD 308 A28838]
RC607.A26A3486   1986   362.1'9697'92   86-21209
ISBN 0-8298-0739-X (pbk.)

The Pilgrim Press, 132 West 31 Street, New York, New York 10001

To all who have suffered
or will suffer as a
consequence of AIDS

Contents

Preface _____

The stories in this book are true. Names and minor details have been changed to obscure identities. The sequence of events and features of particular experiences have not been altered. We have endeavored to tell each person's story faithfully, using his or her language where appropriate and possible. We have refrained from interpreting or commenting about each story or class of subjects until the final chapter. Even in the last chapter we have intentionally refrained from psychoanalyzing stories or any aspect of the AIDS crisis. Rather, the stories and other information provided are an effort to make known to a wider audience the pain, suffering, satisfaction, and peace that people involved with AIDS have experienced and are experiencing. As such, this book is a descriptive and suggestive piece that provides information about a devastating disease, its effect on people (patients and non-patients), the response of society, and the obligation of the church.

The people whose stories are told were carefully selected. We admit a bias in the selection process. Quite intentionally we turned to people whose histories we considered interesting and instructive. Not every category of person with AIDS is represented. For example, no pediatric or solely drug abuse cases are introduced. We are not personally involved with the care of children; and our sample of drug abusers is not large enough to yield an appropriate story. Further, the stories of parents and other family members who totally rejected and abandoned a patient are not here. All these people whom we approached refused to participate in the project. They are seen, however, indirectly in other stories, where their behavior or inaction is reported. Further, noncompliant patients are not represented. Their anger is too overwhelming to allow them to speak instructively. Even so, they are part of the AIDS landscape and their needs ought not to be overlooked. To discern whether their noncompliance is merely emotional or the result of neuropsychiatric factors is difficult at times. Thus, these stories do not present the full spectrum of patients, families, lovers, and health care personnel. The people in these roles who are related to AIDS vary as widely as the people in these roles who are related to any other disease. To generalize on the basis of these stories is tempting, but the temptation should be resisted. The maxim in medicine that "no two patients are alike" holds true in the phenomenon of AIDS; no two persons drawn into the orbit of AIDS are alike. The people who speak in and through this book are representative of their respective populations. They live or work in all parts of the country. It would be a mistake to suppose that everyone is located in or near Houston.

Each person whose story is told was interviewed by one of the authors. One patient's story is told in the first person. The reason for this change in format is given where his story appears. Information derived from one or more of the authors' personal relationships with the person supplements that provided by the interviewee. The use of secondary information was necessary because many people with AIDS cannot recall all that has happened to them, either because there has been so much or because of neurological deficits related to their disease. Our experience with AIDS, the people who suffer with it or as a result of it, and the professional care-providers who struggle to give relief and find a cure suggests that everyone involved has a story. Some stories are heartbreaking, others are heartwarming. None is uninteresting.

We have seen more than 1,000 persons with AIDS or ARC (AIDS-related complex) at the time of this writing. Also, we have come to know countless family members, lovers, and friends. Each individual is unique. Each is affected by us and in turn affects us in a different way. Despite these uniquenesses, we share a common grief that takes many forms and stems from a variety of losses. A colleague accurately described how we feel about our work with AIDS. Emerging from the room of a patient whom he had pronounced dead, he said, "I feel like a soldier in war must feel as he watches his comrades fall one-by-one." He had sojourned with the young man for twenty-four months. His grief was deep and genuine. So is ours and that of everyone else who has been drawn by choice or necessity into the whirl-wind called AIDS.

This book could not have been written without the generous, and at times painful, cooperation of the people whose stories are told on its pages. We are grateful to them for allowing us to invade their privacy and candidly sharing their experiences. We also are indebted to Lolita Cannon, who tolerated numerous interruptions and revisions as she prepared the manuscript. Marion M. Meyer, at The Pilgrim Press, should know of our appreciation for her eager and prompt positive response to our proposal to author this work.

The book is a collaborative effort. The most important collaborators have been the many people touched by AIDS who have taught us about the multiple and varied gains and losses generated by it.

Earl E. Shelp
Ronald H. Sunderland
Peter W.A. Mansell

Houston, Texas

AIDS
and
the Church

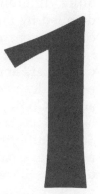

This is a book of stories. To be more accurate, it is a book about people whose lives have been affected by Acquired Immune Deficiency Syndrome (AIDS) or AIDS-Related Complex (ARC). Their stories deserve to be told in order that some of the tragedies associated with AIDS may become known and the necessary resources of the religious and secular communities may be marshaled in compassionate response. The reader will be introduced to people with AIDS or ARC, family members, and lovers whose decisions either to support or to reject affect so gravely the way people with AIDS or ARC cope with their medical crises.

Scientists hope to find a cure in the next five years. It may not come until the next century! Until the breakthrough occurs, AIDS remains a fatal disease, and its course before death brings profound misery to both patients and loved ones. It is something of a miracle, then, that in the face of such trauma there should be any redemptive experiences in the lives of those affected by AIDS. But in the midst of the tragedies, character has emerged, reconciliation has occurred between people who were estranged, and bitterness has given way to acceptance and peace. Tragically, the response is often

1

quite different; some patients are abandoned, condemned by families and friends, and left to die in the company of strangers. The reader will share these experiences in the stories of patients, families, lovers, and care-givers and learn that, in the midst of death, these people deserve and need to experience the love of God and of God's people.

AIDS has become a worldwide public health concern. Some authorities believe that potentially it can have a more devastating effect on humanity than any other disease.[1] Since 1981, the year AIDS was identified, the number of people diagnosed has been doubling at shorter intervals. Its ability to spread rapidly, its fatality, and its insidious complications are responsible for the deep-seated fears, both public and private, that have compounded the suffering of patients and non-patients alike. Initial medical reports concerning the nature and extent of the AIDS epidemic were shrouded in uncertainty. Even now scientists qualify their judgments regarding key elements of the problem: "As far as we know at the moment. . ." This caution, demanded of physicians and scientists involved with AIDS treatment and research, only exacerbates the fear that also has spread like an epidemic across the nation. Researchers have gathered an extraordinary amount of data about AIDS, information that is sufficient to answer many of the initial and subsequent questions. But despite strenuous efforts to correct misinformation and lessen the hysteria with which many people have responded to the disease, many of the early myths have endured and the hysteria continues.

The case of Ryan White, a fourteen-year-old hemophiliac who contracted AIDS through blood products, vividly illustrates the point. In 1985 officials of the school that White attended (Western Middle School in

Kokomo, Indiana) banned him from his seventh-grade classes. While the decision was being appealed in the courts, he received instruction at home by means of a telephone hookup to the classroom. The Indiana Board of Special Education Appeals ordered school officials to request a health certificate from a medical examiner and admit White contingent on this recommendation. On February 13, 1986, a county medical officer ruled that White posed no health threat to classmates or teachers and should be allowed to return to school.

The superintendent of the Western School Corporation was reported to respond: "I don't see any way we can keep Ryan from attending school. That doesn't mean he ought to be there, but I don't think we have any grounds for keeping him out."[2] The response by parents of other children was swift and in total disregard of the overwhelming medical evidence that AIDS is not highly contagious and cannot be contracted through casual contact. Irate parents met in the school auditorium on February 19, 1986, and their ignorance of the medical facts was equalled only by the rampant fear in their words. Television reports showed the angry faces of parents and noted that many parents had acknowledged that they would keep their children home from school the next day. Further, they would seek a court order to ban Ryan from attending school.

This type of reaction was predictable. Many people are incapable of accurately interpreting medical reports about AIDS that are incomplete, simplistic, and oversensationalized. Eye- and ear-catching headlines have politicized a tragic disease and polarized a fearful, ill-informed public. For example, a *New York Times*/CBS News poll indicates that 47 percent of the respondents think that it is possible to contract AIDS by drinking from a glass used by a patient, 32 percent think that the

3

syndrome can be spread through kissing, and 28 percent believe that it is possible to become infected by sitting on a toilet seat used by a person with AIDS.[3] These misunderstandings reinforce fears that have clustered around the appearance of AIDS and compound the pain and suffering of people who are directly or indirectly affected.

First, AIDS evokes a fear of infection and illness. People tend not to become involved in situations where they may be exposed to disease; such behavior would be counterintuitive. It not only would appear ill-advised, but also be considered foolish. People enjoy feeling well, unhindered by illness to pursue work and leisure activities. Only those whose professional commitments involve this level of risk should reasonably be expected to submit to it. For others, infection and its incumbent illness ought to be avoided, perhaps at all costs. The severer an illness, the greater is the sense that any risk of being exposed, either to the infectious agent or to a person believed to be infectious, is too great to assume voluntarily. Because AIDS is an infectious disease that is presently incurable, this fear of infection is greatly intensified. As a result, people with AIDS, or who are believed to have AIDS—or even to be at risk for AIDS—tend to be ostracized and isolated.

Second, public reaction to AIDS has been characterized by a fear of uncertainty. People deny or minimize the fact that nothing in life is free of risk. For example, driving an automobile entails a measurable risk of property damage, injury, and death. Ingesting medication intended to cure entails a degree of risk of failure or may even result in additional trauma to the body. Getting in and out a bathtub entails a statistical risk of injury or death. These types of risk associated with everyday events are appreciated by most people.

4

Nevertheless, they are assumed in order to attain certain goals, for example, moving from one place to another, recovering from illness, or having a clean body. The end, in these instances, is valued more than the risk associated with attaining it.[4] The absence of absolute certainty, or even of the guarantee of reasonable safety, usually does not cause people to avoid customary aspects of contemporary living. In the case of AIDS, however, many people have used the inability of responsible physicians and scientists to issue unqualified assurances regarding infection as a reason to resist exposure to people with AIDS. The uncertainty inherent in these qualified statements evokes a level of fear sufficient to inhibit people from their customary patterns of activities and relationships with respect to this illness. Physical proximity to patients may be shunned. For example, family members may refuse to enter a house or building when an AIDS patient is present. An employer may terminate the employment of a person with AIDS, fearing that his or her continuing involvement will cause clients to take their business elsewhere. When fear caused by uncertainty mounts to levels of hysteria, it becomes demonic, destroying lives and robbing people of both emotional and financial security.

The third form of fear that contributes to an insensitive response to people with AIDS is the fear of death.[5] The association of AIDS with death is unavoidable. Announcements issued by the Centers for Disease Control provide not only the cumulative total of AIDS cases reported, but also the cumulative total of deaths. The perception etched indelibly in the public's mind is that AIDS is a fatal disease. People with AIDS may be seen as the walking dead, the life remaining no longer being considered to count. Thus, to be with a person with AIDS is to be reminded that the patient is terminally ill

5

and that humans are mortal. Even more personally threatening and fearful is the existential reminder that "I" am mortal, that "I" will die. Death is

> The undiscover'd country from whose bourn
> No traveller returns, puzzles the will,
> And makes us rather bear those ills we have
> Than fly to others we know not of.[6]

Death, the unknown, nothingness, separation from the temporal realm in which meaning has been derived, evokes no mere uncertainty, but rather heartfelt fear, the most anxiety-evoking fear of all. This deeply held fear may generate anger that is displaced onto an AIDS patient in whom death is made visible and real.

A fourth form of fear that is heightened by the exploding impact of AIDS is a fear of sexuality and, more specifically, homosexuality. Sexuality evokes great ambivalence. Discussion of sexuality, sexual function, or behavior is often inhibited by personal and societal taboos. Despite medical, anthropological, and religious advances in understanding sexuality, many people hold that it should be clothed in mystery and that sexual contact should conform to archaic societal notions of right and wrong, normal and abnormal, natural and unnatural.[7] People are aware that the outcomes of genital contact may include pregnancy and venereal disease. The former is disvalued outside marriage, and the latter is disvalued under any circumstance. Accordingly, sexual intercourse outside marriage is held to be wrong. The consequences of breaching these social mores often include condemnation and far-reaching disruptions of personal life, family relationships, and professional activity.

Homosexuality and homosexual contact evoke even greater fears because of likely condemnation and recrimination. Homosexual people may be portrayed being deviant, perverted, and, until recently, mentally ill.[8] The stigma attached to homosexuality may engender a fear of homosexual people, lest one be guilty by association, and a fear of one's own homosexual feelings.[9] The association of AIDS with the sexual conduct of gay men reinforces a culturally mediated fear both of sexuality in general and of homosexuality in particular. The potential consequences of AIDS contracted as a result of sexual contact outside marriage (in the case of heterosexual transmission) or homosexual contact are said, by some, to validate traditional proscriptions and legitimate the use of fear as a means of controlling sexual expression. Further, because AIDS is so closely linked to gay men, the faceless threat of AIDS to people is personified in gay men. As a result, fear and anger about AIDS can be translated into fear and anger toward gay men. Thus, people with AIDS and the perceived primary carriers of AIDS are stigmatized and ostracized.

These four fears have converged to constitute an almost unbreakable barrier to rational discussion and development of a humane, sensitive response. One of the most urgent needs is a stronger, more extensive educational program that will make accurate medical facts available to the public. The church has a particularly important role to play in this regard. First, members of congregations, adequately informed, should play a mediating role in their communities. This may well include challenging incorrect information, modeling a balanced response to the crisis in contrast to the prevailing environment of misunderstanding and hysteria, and ministering pastorally to people who are afraid and angry because they fear contagion, as well as to people who are already struggling with the reality of AIDS.

Second, the people of God are called to be a unique

people in society. Their role is to be characterized in terms of community, of service and servanthood, of embodiment of the good news of God's love and the presence of God's reign, and of the reconciling intent of God's love. As the church fulfills these roles, in terms of biblical metaphors, it exists as a sign, a light that shines in a dark world, the savor that adds zest to life, the "first fruits of the kingdom."

Third, the crisis created by AIDS confronts the church with a particular challenge that arises out of the nature of the disease itself and out of the nature of the at-risk population. The church cannot legitimately evade its divine mandate to love and defend oppressed and ostracized people. Words like scourge and plague have been used to compare the impact of AIDS with that of leprosy. People with AIDS understandably resent being identified as "lepers" because of the word's pejorative connotation. AIDS and leprosy are not analogous except in the perception of some members of the public. Nevertheless, because of the perceived similarities, the attitude of Jesus toward lepers in his day can be instructive for the church's response to AIDS in our day. Jesus had fellowship with the lepers, becoming a link between them and the community that excluded them. The example of Father Damien's ministry at the leper colony on Molokai should typify the church's response in such crises. The church's history abounds with similar examples, not the least of which is that of Mother Teresa. Regardless of whether one agrees with her methods, one may respect the motives out of which she is driven to minister to the helpless and forgotten—the poor.

The church's initial response to people with AIDS was, at best, hesitant and ambivalent and, at worst, negligent. Some church leaders have called AIDS God's punishment on homosexual people. Charles Stanley, a

8

former president of the Southern Baptist Convention and a founder of the Moral Majority stated: "God has created the AIDS epidemic to indicate his displeasure over America's acceptance of the homosexual lifestyle."[10] Some Southern Baptist pastors dissociated themselves from Stanley's remarks. Leaders in other churches have been more conciliatory and redemptive. Bishop William E. Swing, Episcopal bishop of California, wrote: "This AIDS crisis is of such gruesome proportions in terms of human suffering that it would be immoral for the church not to enter the arena of pain with thoughtfulness as well as caring."[11] Bishop John R. Quinn called on the Catholic Church in San Francisco "to express our compassion and concern for persons suffering from AIDS, for their families and loved ones. As disciples of Jesus who healed the sick and is Himself the Compassion of God among us, we, too, must show our compassion to our brothers and sisters who are suffering."[12] Mother Teresa established a hospice for people with AIDS in New York City, and a nursing home-residence was founded in Louisville, Kentucky.[13] Finally, the 14th General Synod of the United Church of Christ (1983) adopted an extensive resolution calling for the church to develop special spiritual, educational, and other ministries to all people with AIDS. The 68th General Convention of the Episcopal Church (1985) and the United Methodist Church's General Board of Discipleship (1986) have taken similar actions.

As these latter statements and actions suggest, AIDS raises basic issues of pastoral ministry that are prophetic. They involve the church's role in the community and its responsibility for society's dispossessed. That is, whether or not the federal government or other agencies provide resources to meet the crisis and the needs of people with AIDS, the church must respond in positive, compassionate ways if it is to reflect in its life the spirit of

Jesus, who commanded his fellow servants to do for one another what he had done for them. Many Christians appear to have a problem fulfilling this ministry because the at-risk population mainly consists of gay men and intravenous drug abusers. Both groups are despised and rejected by some Christians, churches, and members of the public. In Old Testament terms, they belong to the category of "the alien in the midst." The Hebrew roots from which "alien" is derived are *ger* (sojourner), *zer* (stranger), and *nakri* (foreigner). These terms apply generally, as the translations suggest, to non-Hebrews residing, often temporarily, in Israel. They were typically traders, travelers, or even soldiers. The moment a stranger entered Israelite territory, he or she came under the full protection of the Law, which dictated that, like others who were deprived of full cultic privileges, the alien's claim on the community for compassionate assistance in adversity was unarguable. The New Testament language is equally compelling. The term foreigner is seldom used. The early Christians considered themselves out of place in the established political and religious arenas of life. They were "aliens" on earth whose service to God and under God was to be directed toward other "aliens," not only fellow believers, but all humanity.[14]

Thomas Ogletree applies the metaphor of the "alien" or "stranger" to the nature of the Christian moral life. He argues that Christian discipleship compels one to be hospitable to the stranger. While acknowledging that a metaphor like "hospitality to strangers" is subject to numerous understandings, Ogletree suggests that it includes at least two basic components: a willingness to protect and an openness to new understandings and experiences.[15] It may even entail joining with the stranger, the vulnerable, and the oppressed in their struggle for liberation, perhaps by being their advocate in places and before powers where their claims for compassion and justice are too often ignored. Contemporary Christians, above all people, should be at home with these images.

As Israel was reminded constantly that it also had been a stranger, and therefore ought to embrace those whose lives were oppressed, so Jesus constantly called his followers to care for the "other." For Israel, the prototypes for the destitute who entreat the community to have regard for their condition were the widow, the orphan, the poor, the stranger at the gate. The Gospel of Matthew adds to this list people who are hungry, thirsty, naked, sick, and imprisoned. But it is the Gospel of Luke that best explicates this duty to befriend and defend the weak. Luke is noted for the emphasis he places on Jesus as the one who speaks for the "poor," the outcast, and the dispossessed, holds them in special regard, and demands of his followers the same measure of compassion. To the Matthean and Lucan lists, it is entirely congruent for the church in the present day to add "the person with AIDS and people in his or her circle." These are people to whom the church has a special obligation.[16]

Christians are commanded to show, not merely to one another but to the neighbor and stranger, that perfect love casts out fear. In the fear-ridden world of AIDS, it is urgent that the love of God revealed in the word and work of Jesus be expressed in works of compassion and ministry by people who bear Jesus' name. Surely, the biblical and theological imperatives directing the church to the "stranger," the "outcast," and the "poor" are well understood and accepted throughout the Christian community. If this is the case, the question must be asked, Why has the church not been more extensively involved in redemptive ministries in response to AIDS? It may be that the reasons for the church's apparent indifference, with an increasing number of notable exceptions, are the same as those that explain the reluctant and inadequate response of governments, other institutions in society, and the general public—fears.

The fears were identified earlier as fears of infection and illness, uncertainty, death, and sexuality. It seems reasonable to imagine that they are operative within congregations as well as within the general public and secular institutions. In addition, the hesitant and measured reaction may be attributable to an unwillingness to risk a more generous and compassionate response being interpreted as an endorsement of the conduct or persons typically associated with AIDS—drug abusers, sexually active people, gay and bisexual men, and prostitutes. This, too, is a form of fear. That this may be the case in churches ought not be surprising. All Christians are not saints. The fears and concerns that they have as finite beings do not disappear automatically or necessarily because of their belief in God or their commitment to Jesus. Nevertheless, the belief and commitment of the people of God ought to be a sufficient motivation to attempt to overcome fears and concerns that stand in the way of true Christian discipleship and legitimate ministry.

The church can turn away from the people who suffer with or as a result of AIDS. Doing so, however, may be costly. The potential costs are intangible for the most part, but they are critical to the life of the church. In short, the church's integrity and credibility are on the line in its response to AIDS. It can be paralyzed by fear, or it can overcome fear to be and do what it is called to be and do.

One way to overcome fear is by education. Education regarding AIDS includes learning what is presently known about the disease, its cause, and its course. These matters are addressed in chapter 2. Also, education regarding AIDS includes learning what it does to people who have the disease, to families and lovers of patients, and to the health care team. These issues are discussed in chapters 3 through 5 as the stories of people in these roles are told. Finally, education includes considering, if not accepting, the observations, perspectives, and experiences of people who have been involved with AIDS and who endeavor to interpret it all from a Christian perspective. This final component of education is presented in the last chapter. Perhaps this form of introduction to and education about AIDS will contribute to a lessening of fear among Christians, and as a result, generate the sort of compassionate, supportive, and redemptive ministries that are required by AIDS.

Medical Facts About AIDS

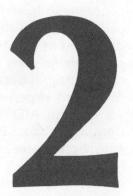

Early in 1981 some physicians in southern California reported the occurrence of a then uncommon form of pneumonia, *Pneumocystis carinii* pneumonia (PCP), in a small group of gay males. The interest of the medical and scientific communities was not aroused, however, until a number of cases of a rare variety of cancer, Kaposi's sarcoma, was reported soon thereafter in a similar group of male homosexuals in the New York City area.[1] *P. carinii* pneumonia is an opportunistic infection; it is caused by an organism (*P. carinii*) that probably inhabits the lungs and tissues of most normal people without causing any clinical disease. In people with compromised immune systems, PCP is often fatal. People most at risk are those who have an impaired immune system, for example, very young, malnourished children, the aged, and individuals whose immune systems have been compromised, either as a result of medical treatment or by some other cause.

Before 1981 Kaposi's sarcoma was seen in less than 500 individuals annually in the United States. This uncommon tumor was first described in 1879 by an Austro-Hungarian dermatologist, Moriz Kohn, who later changed his name to Moriz Kaposi.[2] Kaposi's sarcoma occurred most commonly in its so-called classical form in people who were in their sixties and seventies, usually men, and who were of eastern Mediterranean origins. The disease progresses slowly, seldom causing death. Its lesions are predominantly seen on the ankles and feet. The endemic form has been common in countries in central and western Africa (e.g., Zaire, Ruanda-Burundi, Uganda, Kenya, Chad). In these countries the disease spreads more rapidly, tends to affect people in their twenties and thirties, again predominantly male, but often involves parts of the body other than the skin, such as the gastrointestinal tract, bone, brain, lungs, and, particularly, lymph nodes. The endemic form also is called the lymphadenopathic form of Kaposi's sarcoma. It has been suggested that the endemic form of Kaposi's sarcoma may have as one of the possible causative agents the herpesvirus or cytomegalovirus (CMV), although this has never been proved.

Kaposi's sarcoma occurs in people who have been artificially immunosuppressed, for instance, after an organ transplant (e.g., kidney, heart). Some transplant recipients receiving immunosuppressive drugs, which prevent the body's immune response from rejecting the donor organ, will develop a malignancy, the most common being one of the lymphomas, followed by Kaposi's sarcoma. In some cases when administration of the immune suppressive drug is discontinued, the Kaposi's lesions spontaneously disappear.

The number of people with Kaposi's sarcoma or opportunistic infections increased rapidly after 1981. It was soon recognized that most individuals affected by what came to be called Acquired Immune Deficiency Syndrome (AIDS) were young male homosexuals whose average age was approximately thirty-two years. It also became clear that other people were affected by the disease—intravenous drug users, a small number of

15

hemophiliacs, some individuals who had blood transfusions, and a number of recent Haitian immigrants. As data were gathered, it was hypothesized that a transmissible agent, probably viral, was the cause of AIDS. Evidence supporting this hypothesis included its epidemiological features, its clustered occurrence around the United States, and data suggesting a geographical spread from California and the New York-New Jersey area to other parts of the country and the world (e.g., Canada and Europe).

As unusual infections and Kaposi's sarcoma, separately or together, were reported during 1981 and 1982, it was evident that a new situation had emerged. The common factors were that (a) the patients were predominantly young, gay males and (b) all of them had evidence of immunological abnormalities, particularly in the set of lymphocytes called T cells and, more specifically, the helper T cell subset. Investigations into this phenomenon revealed that these abnormalities were far more wide-ranging than had been thought, including abnormalities in skin test reactivity, in the absolute number of helper cells, and in the ratio of helper-suppressor cells. Abnormalities were also found in the B, or antibody-producing, cells and in other cells of the cellular immune system, called macrophages. Immunocompromised patients were unable to respond adequately to a number of new situations, such as infections and malignant diseases.[3]

P. carinii pneumonia and Kaposi's sarcoma were not the only complications of AIDS. A number of other opportunistic infections, caused by fungi, protozoa, bacteria, and viruses, also were seen.[4] Similarly, lymphomas[5] and ordinary carcinomas, such as those of the oropharynx and the anorectal area, were reported. Investigations into the immunological abnormalities seen with AIDS uncovered many additional problems that the AIDS patient experienced: an inability to mount immune responses to new infectious agents, already encountered viral and other infectious agents, and increased levels of gamma globulins and immune complexes. It was as if the affected individual's entire immunological apparatus had become unhinged and unable to respond either to preexisting or new challenges.

The number of cases reported in the United States and in many other parts of the world continued to increase. Epidemiological studies suggested that some features were characteristic in most individuals affected with the disease; they tended to be relatively young male homosexuals who led a fast-track existence, having multiple, often anonymous, sexual partners, and they appeared to have a high incidence of recreational drug use, particularly of inhaled nitrites.[6] Anal intercourse and other anal manipulations were common practices of affected individuals. A study conducted in 1982 indicated that the receptive partner of anal intercourse was at higher risk for AIDS, giving rise to a theory that the transmissible agent, whatever it was, could be passed in seminal fluid and enter the bloodstream after the trauma that often results from anal intercourse.[7] Other infections—a history of syphilis, gonorrhea, hepatitis B, cytomegalovirus and Epstein-Barr virus infections, to name only a few—often occurred concomitantly with AIDS.[8]

In 1983 researchers at the Institute Pasteur in Paris isolated a virus, which they named lymphadenopathy virus (LAV), from the enlarged lymph node of an individual suffering from AIDS.[9] It belonged to the RNA (ribonucleic acid) group of viruses known as retroviruses. Members of this family cause malignant disease in animals. The French scientists were unable to produce large amounts of the virus for study, mainly because a suitable culture system was not known at the time. For this and other reasons, the discovery went largely unrecognized by the rest of the scientific and medical world. Almost exactly a year later a similar virus was isolated in laboratories at the National Institutes of Health in the United States. This time, fortunately, a culture system was available, making extensive study of the virus possible. The virus was named HTLV-III (human T lymphocyte virus, type III), HTLV-I and II being viruses known to affect the lymphocyte system of white blood cells and cause lymphoma and leukemia. One of the striking features of HTLV-III was that it seemed preferentially to infect the helper T cell system, the system of immunologically active lymphocytes that is both quantitatively and qualitatively abnormal in AIDS.[10]

At approximately the same time, workers in San Francisco isolated a virus called AIDS Related Virus (ARV), which proved to be virtually identical to both LAV and HTLV-III.[11] Much is now known about this virus with several names. It infects T helper cells, B cells, and macrophages. The body is capable of producing antibodies to it, although these antibodies do not seem to provide protection. An infection is extremely long lasting and is seldom, if ever, cleared naturally from an infected individual. The effect that the AIDS virus has on the immune system is analogous to shooting the conductor of an orchestra during a performance. The conductor is the T helper lymphocyte and the remainder of the orchestra represents the other immunological defense mechanisms. Depending on the state of training of the orchestra, in this case the health of the individual, the orchestra may be able to continue for a variable length of time after the conductor is removed, but eventually it will break down and be unable to perform coherently. This is exactly what happens in AIDS; the central actor, or conductor, of the immunological orchestra is the helper cell without whose presence the remainder of the orchestra will gradually fail and become ineffective.

The virus, by itself, is not responsible for the occurrence of Kaposi's sarcoma, malignancies associated with AIDS, or the opportunistic infections. It is simply responsible for the immunological abnormalities. Many individuals may be infected with this virus but probably will never develop full-blown AIDS. This fact is of extreme importance when one realizes that other cofactors are also operating. These cofactors, such as sexually transmitted diseases, recreational drugs, malnutrition, and some life-style attributes, are largely avoidable. Thus, it should be emphasized that AIDS is, to some extent, a preventable, or at least avoidable, disease.

Once the virus was recognized and characterized, it was hoped that a vaccine would be the next step. However, because the virus exists in many forms and can change spontaneously, producing a vaccine is a difficult task. Not only does the virus infect the cells of the immunological system, but those of the central nervous system as well.[12] This has serious consequences, since once a nerve cell is destroyed it never regenerates. Also, because of the existence of the blood-brain barrier, the chance that an antiviral drug, should one be discovered, could penetrate effectively into the brain is not particularly good. One of the tragic consequences of infection by the AIDS virus is that the individual very early in the course of the disease may suffer a number of distressing and permanent, slowly progressive neurological defects, ranging from short-term memory loss and changes in affect to dementia and paralysis.

Early in the recognition of this syndrome it was clear that a clinical condition existed that did not satisfy the strict Centers for Disease Control criteria for AIDS. People with this condition, originally called AIDS prodrome, were in groups at high risk of getting AIDS and exhibited a number of signs and symptoms associated with full-blown AIDS: fever, weight loss, diarrhea, night sweats, fatigue, and swollen lymph nodes. They also showed a greater or lesser degree of immunological abnormality and evidence of infection by the AIDS virus. However, they are not troubled, as of yet, by opportunistic infections or one of the cancers characteristic of the syndrome. The condition is now called AIDS-related complex (ARC).[13] Because AIDS is a reportable disease, the number of people diagnosed can be somewhat readily known. ARC is not presently a reportable disease. It is not known, therefore, how many people are affected. The number of persons with ARC is estimated to be at least ten times, if not a hundred times, greater than the number of persons with AIDS. Nor is it known how many individuals with ARC will develop full-blown AIDS.[14] Current estimates range from 10 to 25%. Further, no one knows how long it will take for these individuals to develop AIDS. It may be a 25% absolute risk. In other words, 25% of the ARC population will develop AIDS during their lifetime. Alternatively, it may be a 25% annual risk; that is, each year 25% of the ARC population will develop AIDS. If the risk is annual, every person with ARC ultimately will develop AIDS.

Current estimates of the number of persons infected by the AIDS virus also vary. On the one hand, it may be that as few as one-half million persons are infected. On the other hand, it may be that more than 2 million persons are infected. Although it is impossible to be certain, the higher number appears to be more accurate. For example, in California, where surveys to determine the number of infected persons have been conducted with some degree of care, it is thought that between 350,000 and 500,000 persons are infected in that state alone. It seems reasonable, if the California estimates are accurate, that the number of infected persons in the remaining forty-nine states would push the national total at least to the higher of the two estimates.

Another area of uncertainty is the incubation period of the disease. It varies with the age and immunological status of the patient and the amount of virus transferred. Thus, if an infant is exposed to a large dose of virus, the incubation period may be relatively short. If, however, an adult is infected as a result of one or a small number of exposures after sexual intercourse, the incubation period may be quite long, possibly seven or even ten years. Even though the virus' incubation period is uncertain, it has a relatively low infectivity, being not nearly as infectious, for instance, as smallpox, influenza, or hepatitis B. For example:

> If you draw one cubic centimeter of blood—about enough to fill an eyedropper—from a person who's infected with the tenacious and widespread virus that causes hepatitis B, put it into a swimming pool containing 24,000 gallons of water, extract a cubic centimeter of water from the pool and inject it into a chimpanzee, there will be enough virus in the shot to infect the chimp. But if you put the same amount of blood from someone who's infected with the AIDS virus into the pool, if the chlorine in the water didn't kill it (which it almost certainly would), the virus wouldn't infect a chimp—or anyone else. Even if you diluted the virus in only a quart of water, the chances of giving a chimp AIDS with a one-cc shot of that water would be about one in ten.[15]

In short, and to state it bluntly, one has to work hard to be infected with the AIDS virus.

Much is also known about the means by which the

virus is transmitted. There is, for instance, no evidence that the virus can be transmitted by social or casual contact or by such agents as rodents or mosquitos. Large-scale studies conducted in families of children with AIDS have shown no evidence of the virus being transmitted from one individual to another by such activities as kissing, hugging, using the same utensils or crockery, or merely living in the same general area as an affected person. Further, there is no risk of contracting the disease as a result of contamination by food handlers, hairdressers, or florists or by contact with any number of other occupations often associated with high-risk groups. Similarly, there is no danger to school-children from contact with a child with AIDS, unless that child habitually exhibits behavior such as vicious biting or inability to control bladder or bowel movements. Nor is there any risk with respect to the use of the common cup in eucharistic celebrations.

The only known way in which the AIDS virus can be transmitted is by direct introduction into a recipient's bloodstream. This may occur by using infected needles, in the case of intravenous drug abusers, or as a result of transfusion of blood or blood products. A number of serological tests for antibodies against the AIDS virus recently have become available. These are currently administered in all blood banks and at a number of alternate sites around the country. Every blood donor has his or her serum tested for the presence of antibody against the virus. If antibodies are found, the donated unit of blood is discarded and the donor is informed that the confirmatory test is positive.

The antibody test suffers from a number of drawbacks, since a small proportion, probably considerably less than one percent, will be false positives. In other words, individuals will test positive though not having evidence of the relevant antibodies in their blood. Such persons may be suffering from one of a variety of auto-immune diseases. There also will be a small, but uncertain, number of false negatives—individuals who have been in contact with the AIDS virus but, for one reason or another, do not have measurable antibody levels. Their exposure may be too recent for antibodies to be produced, or alternatively they have not produced enough antibodies for a relatively insensitive test to identify. These false results will continue to be a problem until a more accurate test is devised. Despite these minor problems in testing, the U.S. blood-banking system is much safer now that the antibody test is available. There is no reason for people who need blood transfusions to refuse an immediate life-saving intervention because of the remote possibility of contracting AIDS by this means.

The virus also can be transmitted from men to women and from women to men by heterosexual intercourse. This mode of transmission seems to be dominant in central and western African countries, such as Zaire, Ruanda, and Uganda, where the incidence of the disease is much higher than in the United States. For instance, in Zaire, the incidence of the disease is approximately 100 per 100,000 population. In the capital city of Kinshasa, with a population of 3 million, this should result in 3,000 cases per annum. Also, Zaire's male-female ratio is approximately 1:1, whereas in the United States less than one in ten AIDS patients is a woman. Also of concern in the African situation is the high level of serum positivity to the AIDS virus in pediatric patients admitted to hospital in Kinshasa.[16] The rate currently is about 9%. AIDS in children may result from infection by the use of contaminated needles. Alternatively, these children may have been infected by their mothers while in the womb. Depending upon a variety of factors, these children may develop the disease during infancy or later in childhood. It is not possible to be precise about the situation in Africa, although it seems certain that the disease has been common in that area for much longer than it has in the United States. Whether in the African experience we are looking at the future, in the sense that this ultimately will be the situation in the United States, is not known at present. It is hypothesized that the disease probably occurred in Africa as a result of the passage of a similar virus from African green monkeys into humans. Further, the disease may have appeared in the United States as a result of transmission from western Africa to Haiti, by Haitians either working in Zaire or accompanying Cuban forces invading Angola. It was brought back to the Caribbean basin, transmitted to American homosexuals vacationing in Haiti, and then spread to other parts of the world.

The treatment of AIDS and AIDS-related complications is difficult. There are some relatively successful therapies for Kaposi's sarcoma and the other malignancies, although complete remission is uncommon, and the length of the remission is short. One of the big problems is that such methods as chemotherapy carry the added danger of further decreasing the immune capabilities of a patient whose immune system is already greatly compromised. Therefore, although the remission rates of the actual malignancy may be quite high, the possibility of increasing the risk of a fatal infection is also high. Treatment of Kaposi's sarcoma currently relies either on the use of small doses of chemotherapeutic drugs designed to have minimal toxicity and maximum efficiency or on the use of such agents as interferon in combination with chemotherapy or other biological response modifiers.

Therapy for opportunistic infections is relatively standard except that many of the diseases afflicting AIDS patients are difficult, if not impossible, to treat.[17] *P. carinii* pneumonia, the most common opportunistic infection in AIDS patients, has an approximately 60 percent cure rate on the first infection but carries a high recurrence rate of around 30 percent. Standard treatment (co-trimoxazole [Bactrim]) can be complicated by a high percentage of allergic reactions, necessitating the use of another drug (pentamidine), which has toxic side effects of its own, thus complicating the continued use of maintenance doses for prophylaxis. Other therapeutic agents have shown some efficacy (Dapsone, DFMO), but all may have toxic side effects and none improves the underlying immunodeficiency that allows opportunistic infections to occur.

A great effort has been put into the study of drugs designed specifically to modulate the immune system. However, none so far has been generally effective. This is because treating an AIDS patient with a biological response modifier is like pouring water into a bucket with a hole in the bottom. In this illustration the hole is produced by the virus, which continues to destroy the immune system and may, in some cases, do so even faster in the presence of some agents that increase the number of cells in which the virus lives. Although such agents as Isoprinosine, interleukin 2, and a large number of others have been claimed to be effective in reversing the immune destruction in AIDS, there is no conclusive evidence at this point that they influence the clinical course of AIDS. A central issue in treatment is the production and use of an effective antiviral drug. A number of such drugs—suramin, ribavirin, azimathymidine, to name a few—are currently available and under investigation. Clinical trials are in the early stages. Not enough is known about any of these agents to say with certainty that one or more represent the answer to the problem. In any case, combination treat-

ments of antiviral and immune restorative agents probably will prove to be the solution in the long term. Until
then, the medical treatment of people with AIDS and
ARC will be provisional. The number of untimely
deaths will continue to grow. The life expectancies of
people with ARC will remain indeterminate and people
with AIDS can expect to live, on average, about two
years after diagnosis. The economic costs will skyrocket
(estimated to be $6.2 billion for the first 10,000 cases of
AIDS in the United States[18]), and the costs in human
pain and suffering will remain incalculable.

As a closing comment on the treatment of AIDS, the
malignancies, and the devastating infections often seen
in patients, Murphy's laws numbered 1, 2, 4, 5, and 7
are descriptive and predictive:

1. If anything can go wrong, it will.
2. Nothing is ever as simple as it seems.
4. If there is a possibility of several things going
   wrong, the first to go wrong will be the one that
   will do the most damage.
5. Left to themselves, things go from bad to worse.
7. If everything seems to be going well, you obviously have overlooked something.

In summary, AIDS is a new disease characterized by
profound abnormalities in cell-mediated immunity, the
consequences of which are an increased incidence of
some previously uncommon forms of malignancy and
opportunistic infections. The cause of AIDS seems
clearly to be a virus (HTLV-III/LAV/ARV—now generally
referred to as HIV [human immunodeficiency virus]),
although a number of cofactors are contributory. Because of the peculiar circumstances of AIDS patients,
treatment of the malignancies and opportunistic infections is complicated, demanding, on the one hand,

treatment not likely to compromise the immune system further and, on the other, extreme urgency to respond quickly to infectious diseases. The most logical and likely cure will be a combination of antiviral and immune restorative measures. One consequence of being able to achieve this in AIDS is that it might also be possible to prevent other malignant and infectious diseases by reconstituting an individual's immune system. Finally, the rate at which AIDS will spread in the homosexual, drug abuse, and heterosexual communities depends on numerous conditions, some of which are avoidable or preventable. After years of study and observation, it is safe to conclude that the general public ought not be inordinately concerned about infection from the routine conduct of daily life. Neither should people be reluctant to minister routinely to people with AIDS or ARC. Casual contact with patients presents no known risk for infection by the AIDS virus. For more intimate ministries, such as nursing care, appropriate precautions are indicated as a matter of prudence. Given these considerations, people with this disease need not be isolated from the public, worship, work, family, or friends.

Quite apart from the clinical manifestations of AIDS, many social, ethical, philosophical, theological, economic, and legal problems surround the disease. Some of these are illustrated in the stories that follow in the next three chapters.

People with AIDS or ARC

3

JIM

Jim lived in the fast lane of gay life. He liked to "party." Many weekday and most weekend nights were spent in cruise or dance bars. Standing 6½ feet tall and weighing 230 pounds, Jim stood out in the crowd. He was proud of his size. Workouts at a gym were a routine part of his weekly schedule. In short, Jim was "tall, dark, and handsome." These physical attributes were important resources that he could use to obtain the level of attention and affirmation that he thought he needed.

Jim was born and grew up in Chicago. His mother and father divorced when he was three years old. Although the wages his mother earned as a cashier were meager, she did what she could to provide for him. For two years after his parents' divorce, Jim's home was his mother's car. He amused himself in the car as best he could during the day while his mother worked. Jim's situation improved some when his mother remarried. The car that had been his home for two years was left behind. Jim had a new place to live and a new father. The former he considered a gain; the latter turned out to be a disaster. His stepfather was a huge man, weighing about 350 pounds, or so it seemed to Jim when he would sit on Jim as he was forced to lie on the floor with his arms crossed over his chest. Jim thought that this was his stepfather's abusive way of establishing his authority over Jim. Jim never told his mother about these episodes. He coped with the abuse as well as he could. But when he was old enough he enlisted in the army, leaving high school, stepfather, and mother behind.

Jim never fully adjusted to life as a soldier. After eighteen months he was discharged because of his homosexual conduct and abuse of drugs and alcohol. Freed from home and the military, Jim set out to see the great cities of the nation—at least the gay parts of them. His pilgrimage took him to New York City, San Francisco, Miami, and Houston. Jim always looked at men sexually. Male bodies fascinated him; female bodies didn't. As early as his eighth year he wondered what it would be like to have sex with a man. He felt drawn to older, more experienced men who could teach him sexually. He was successful sexually, having between eight and fifteen partners a week. He was not successful, however, in maintaining relationships. Jim had three lovers after he left home. The first relationship ended after three years. The second lasted for two years. The third ended after sixty-five days, when Jim died of complications of AIDS.

Jim's family knew that he was gay. His sexuality was never condemned by his mother. She did object to, but said little about, his intravenous drug abuse. Drugs were a big part of Jim's life. They not only allowed him to feel better about himself, but were also the cement of the relationships he had with his bar-based friends. He tried to maintain employment apart from gay bars and sex-related businesses but was not successful. His use of amphetamines and alcohol always seemed to get in the way.

Drugs became a source of income. Jim found that he could make more money selling drugs than by working a regular daytime job. The profits from drugs grew as he found jobs in settings where he could have more direct contact with his primary market of fast-lane gay men. He worked as a disc jockey in gay dance bars for seven and a half years and as a clerk in an adult bookstore for one year. Both settings were conducive to his drug sales and his desire to be immersed in a segment of gay culture.

When Jim became ill his drug-related and sex-based friends disappeared. He must have intuitively expected this response. Early indications in 1983 that he might be ill were ignored and kept secret. A persistent cough, night sweats, weight loss, and deteriorating eyesight were rationalized to be something else, even though he knew what they probably meant. The symptoms and diseases associated with AIDS were well known to Jim. After all, by 1983 the disease had already claimed the lives of about twenty gay men that he knew, including his first lover. But when he found the first lesion on his skin indicative of Kaposi's sarcoma, he went to a physician to have his suspicions confirmed.

Jim's battle with AIDS lasted for twenty months. Alcohol and recreational drugs were left behind as prescribed drugs to combat his many illnesses took their place. His kitchen counter looked like a small, well-stocked pharmacy. These agents and the professional care that he received became his source of hope and connections to life. The bars, bookstores, and buddies that filled his life before gradually were replaced by clinics, hospital rooms, doctors, nurses, forms, and a few loyal friends. And as he fought to live, the death toll of people that he knew increased to more than forty. The many funerals and memorial services that he attended started to make him "crazy." With each one he speculated about when his time to die would come. Yet, despite these deaths, nine hospitalizations, and other losses, Jim wanted to live.

Jim told his mother that he had been diagnosed as having AIDS. Her response was particularly pleasing. She wrote him a letter encouraging him to fight, reminding him that they had survived many hardships, including the two years that they lived in her car. She recalled that the popular song, "You and Me Against the World," recorded by Helen Reddy, had been *their* song during difficult days. He was encouraged to persevere now as they had persevered before. And for the first time in Jim's memory, his mother told him that she loved him. He always thought that she did, but somehow she seemed unable before then to say the words.

Jim visited his mother and stepfather in Chicago once after he was diagnosed. It wasn't a totally rewarding experience. The visit was aborted soon after Jim was served a meal on a paper plate and given plastic utensils to use. Hurt and angry, Jim returned to Houston, vowing not to go home again. His mother continued to contact Jim during the rest of his life. She came to Houston twice during hospitalizations that Jim was not expected to survive. Their relationship was restored as a result of her initiatives. As Christmas 1985 approached, Jim was looking forward to her visit. He knew, however, that his life was fading away. On Thanksgiving Day he remarked, "If Mom doesn't come soon, she won't get to say good-bye to Jim."

Jim never regretted, nor felt guilty about, being gay. And after feeling initially that having AIDS was unfair, he came to view it as "the best thing that ever happened to me." His addiction to methamphetamines was broken. He finally heard his mother say to him, "I love you." He had a lover relationship based on something other than drugs or sex. And because of what he experi-

31

enced, he developed a concern for the welfare of other gay men. He spoke to gay men during seminars designed to instruct them about safe sex practices. He gave interviews to the local media, describing what it was like to have AIDS, to watch one's body weight decrease 100 pounds, to be isolated, feared, and stigmatized, to gradually grow weaker and become totally dependent on other people. Jim enjoyed the attention, but he grieved the many losses that were the reasons for it.

His disease and the response of people to it forced Jim to reconsider what is important in life. His relationship with his final lover, a young man who loved Jim without expecting anything in return, became an incentive to live. Jim was a demanding patient, seeking and needing almost constant attention as he approached his final illness. Bart, Jim's lover, was a small man, weakened by illnesses associated with AIDS-related complex (ARC) and by the level of care that Jim required. It was a mighty struggle for Bart, 5 feet 8 inches tall and weighing approximately 120 pounds, to lift Jim from bed to wheelchair and back. Jim felt that this level of dependency was dehumanizing. At times he thought about hastening the death that he knew was inevitable. After all, one of his best friends who had AIDS killed himself by injecting street drugs into his catheter. When in depressed moods Jim would say of his friend, "Son-of-a-bitch, he left me here. He should have taken me with him." Nevertheless, despite his physical pain and emotional losses, Jim clung to life, Bart, and the few other relationships that made life worth living.

Jim never cared much for the church. He attended a Roman Catholic school for the first and second grades. His expulsion for being a "holy terror" was the beginning of his estrangement and antipathy toward organized religion, which he considered a "bunch of bullshit." Jim thought that the "pomp, icons, and gold" were the main interests of the church, rather than "spirituality" or "the search for God." Jim believed that there is a God, a higher power, who helped him to get over his addictions to alcohol and drugs. This same power, Jim believed, could help him to cope with or overcome AIDS. Orthodox theology and Christian moral condemnations were rejected by Jim. AIDS was not God's judgment on him or anyone else, according to Jim. His God cared for him now and would provide for him beyond death in a realm without hurt or pain, where love and compassion are more abundant than on earth.

Jim believed that he had always been searching for God, for a spiritual awakening, throughout his life. AIDS, in his mind, had enabled him to find God, to be awakened spiritually. The God in whom Jim believed was found in the midst of his experience with AIDS. He began to have a sense of completion or wholeness. His life, and life in general, somehow began to make sense. In a way that Jim could not understand or articulate, AIDS made him a person, able to separate the important from the trivial. AIDS forced him to turn away from a life of constant partying. The fair-weather friends that he had were left behind. AIDS had brought some people together into more meaningful relationships, including him and Bart. The experience of these more meaningful relationships was part of what Jim meant when he spoke of searching for and having a spiritual awakening. These relationships, and the mutual commitments that sustained them, were what Jim thought he would take with him into "the next life" that he entered in November 1985 at the age of twenty-eight years.

SCOTT

Scott, a gifted musician, discovered that he was gay during his teenage years. His parents were leaders in a conservative congregation in a small city in Arkansas. Scott felt that they would not understand his sexuality so he never told them. He simply did not want to hurt them. He was baptized during his youth, as is the custom in his denomination, but didn't experience a "change of heart" until 1974. Between his youth and conversion he attended worship but felt uneasy about how God viewed his homosexual activity. His discomfort, however, was not sufficient to cause him to forego the pleasures of sexual encounters with men before or after 1974.

Scott's homosexuality was not the only secret in his life. He never told his aging parents and brother that he had ARC. They were told that he had a rare blood disorder that was not responding to treatment. His parents and brother wanted to visit him, but they were asked not to do so. Once again, Scott wanted to protect them from seeing him in his deteriorating condition. Their daily phone calls, and financial support after he became unable to work, were vital sources of hope and comfort.

He was intelligent, witty, outgoing, generous, selfless, and gracious. He graduated from college with a degree in communication arts. After college he worked for twenty years as a disc jockey at one radio station or another. During his career as a radio personality he began to work as a pianist at an exclusive hotel. Playing piano and having an immediate rapport with people were more satisfying to Scott than talking into a microphone. His radio career was slowly set aside in favor of his work as a musician and entertainer. He worked alone until he met a talented young man who played violin.

Scott met John in a gay bar. John worked at the bar picking up bottles and glasses. He came to Houston in 1980 to be treated for a dependency on alcohol and drugs that developed after he divorced his wife. Being in a heterosexual marriage didn't mean that he wasn't gay. He was in a gay relationship for six years before he married. John's parents knew of his homosexuality. They didn't understand why John married. In retrospect, neither does he. Nevertheless, his parents tried to accept each of his partners. All that they wanted was for John to be happy. The happiness that they desired for him finally was found when he met Scott.

As Scott and John talked on the first night they met, they discovered each other's interest in music. Their conversation lasted until closing time. Scott offered to drive John home. John refused, explaining that he slept on the pool table in the bar. They agreed, however, that John would visit Scott the next day so that they could play music together.

As they played the next day, John's training, experience, and talent impressed Scott. Soon afterward John became Scott's roommate. They grew together as friends, never sexual partners. John looks back at Scott's invitation as providential. It literally saved John from a life on the streets. It meant also that the facts about Scott's life that he never wanted his family to know could be kept secret. They grew to love each other. And as Scott became ill, he never feared that John would not be there to take care of him or be with him when he died.

Like Jim, but not to the same degree, Scott enjoyed alcohol, drugs, and men. His wit and charm, together with his nicely proportioned body, enabled him to be sexually active until he began to be ill. Scott vacationed in Florida in 1981. Soon after returning home he developed a viral infection that mostly kept him in bed for six months. He resumed his usual routine of work and socializing after he recovered. But he never truly felt good again. At first his physician wasn't able to tell him

35

what was wrong. As time passed and he had recurrent episodes of illness, it was determined that he had ARC. The main manifestations were chronic diarrhea, yeast infections (candidiasis), and chronic hepatitis. From 1981 to 1985 Scott's condition worsened. His weight dropped from 167 pounds to 115 pounds. He became unable to work. He knew what was happening to him. His objective was to make the best of it.

Like most people with ARC, Scott never progressed to a diagnosis of AIDS. Unlike most people with ARC, Scott expected to die of his disease. He grew weaker and incontinent. Nevertheless, he maintained a cheerful spirit until the end. His concern for John never lessened. His interest in the well-being of clinic personnel never failed. The physicians and nurses who watched him decline over forty-eight months had become his friends. They went to hear him, John, and a third colleague perform. They had lunch together. Gradually they developed the sort of relationship that led his primary physician to feel deep pain resulting from an inability to help.

The grief experienced by Scott's physician was not shared by Scott. As noted earlier, Scott became a Christian in 1974. Even though he continued to engage in homosexual conduct, somehow he reconciled his life and behavior with his religious beliefs. His illness, or any adversity, happened for a reason. He didn't speculate about why he was ill. Somehow he was at peace with himself and God about being gay, ill, and dying. He looked forward to death, confident that John, whom he regarded as a son, would be with him.

This does not mean that Scott did not grieve the loss of certain abilities and unrealized dreams. He dearly missed playing the piano. He knew, as well, that his desire to move with John to New Mexico would never be fulfilled. They had planned to build and live in a log cabin, playing and writing music together. But his body weakened. His pain grew more intense. Death was approaching.

Late in 1984, ten years after his "change of heart," Scott decided that he had to come to terms with God about his homosexuality. He did this alone, calling on his religious training as a child and the beliefs that he internalized from Sunday morning services. Scott and John worshiped almost every Sunday at a large, fundamentalist, Protestant church. John joined the church soon after meeting Scott. John's baptism and subsequent participation in the church's music ministry were sources of pride for Scott. Although both Scott and John occasionally had sex with other men, they were unconvinced that it was right. They turned to scripture for guidance. They jointly decided that "no practicing homosexuals would be in heaven." As a result, both became celibate in 1984, even though Scott had become a Christian in 1974 and John had become a Christian in 1981.

Scott prayed while he lay in bed. He prayed for the salvation of his friends. He asked God to do what was best for him. He never asked God to take him. God would do that when it was time. Scott was willing to be patient. His illness had allowed him to become closer to God before he died. He appreciated the time and the opportunity that God gave him. Death would be a relief. He was not afraid. The anticipation and peace with which he approached death came, according to him, from an "inner joy that he had conformed his life to what the Bible teaches." He looked forward to "being with Jesus." Both he and John would be freed with his death. Scott would be freed from pain. John would be freed to resume his musical career and life.

Despite his willingness to die, Scott wanted to live until December 14. The Christmas pageant at the church where he and John worshiped was scheduled for this night. John had been rehearsing with the orchestra for weeks. Scott dearly wanted to attend this event. After this he was "ready for anything." Unfortunately, he died at home six days before the scheduled performance. Scott did what he wished would happen. He simply rolled over in his bed and "went to sleep" with a smile on his face. John was with him, as Scott knew that he would be. His secrets had been kept from his family. Scott's life was over after forty-six years. John's began again, after a two-year interruption of devoted service to Scott, at the age of thirty-four.

GARY

Gary is the sort of person who seems unable to feel good about himself. He never seems to fit in anywhere for very long. His parents wanted their marriage, family, and home to be perfect. Unfortunately, Gary wasn't perfect. In stereotypical middle-class fashion, he was sent to a psychiatrist who, according to Gary, wanted him to be the therapeutic catalyst for the whole family. He has tried over the years to satisfy everyone, to comply with their wishes for him, and not to create a disruption. His sole goal in life has been to please people. Instead of being affirmed for this manner of living, this soft-spoken, unsophisticated, sincere man has become the human carpet that everyone walks on.

Gary's family lived in Pennsylvania until he was eighteen years old. During his childhood and adolescence Gary always felt "inclined toward men." Everything about men seemed to fascinate him—their bodies, the way they walked, their mannerisms, their interests. He did not make the connection of his interest in men to his awakening homosexuality until he was sixteen years old.

His sixteenth year was revelatory. First, he was told that his father was actually his stepfather. Gary remembered being at a wedding ceremony involving his mother as the bride when he was four years old. He had never questioned anyone about this memory. As far as he was concerned it was a second ceremony in which his mother and father affirmed their original vows. He wondered why the truth had been kept from him for so long. Also, the deception caused him to wonder about his place in the family. Second, Gary tried out for a part in a play at his high school. He thought that it would be a fun thing to do. His mother was infuriated when Gary told her of his interest in theater. She strongly proclaimed that she didn't want her son to be an actor, hairdresser, decorator, or florist. Again, Gary wasn't able to make the presumed connection between these occupations and homosexuality. It seemed to him that his mother simply disapproved of his interest and him. Feeling unwanted and out of place, Gary took his guitar and ran away to New York City.

Gary decided to stay at a YMCA in New York. He was propositioned in an elevator by an older man. They went to the man's room, where they had sex. Gary felt good about what happened. In his words, "it was too much fun not to do it again." He didn't have to wait long. After a week in New York he returned to his hometown. He was picked up at the train station by two men who were lovers. He stayed with them for two weeks before returning home.

Little was said when he returned home. The same disinterest in him that he felt before remained. His parents would tell him to come to them for a talk if he had a problem. But then when he would try to tell them how he felt, they wouldn't listen. They were, according to Gary, emotionally closed to him, and perhaps to each other, since Gary has no memory of seeing them touch or kiss. His efforts to talk to them seemed always to result in an argument. It was never convenient for them to deviate from their concerted drive for middle-class respectability to help their son, who was searching for himself and evidence of their love for him. His problems, in their view, were "molehills" compared with their concerns, which were "mountains." By the time he moved out of his parents' home, Gary had learned a lesson: the way to deal with adversity is to be cold, strong, and dispassionate.

Gary's negative feelings about himself have endured through the years. When his family moved to Texas he went away to attend college for one year. He never returned to school. The world and work were seen as new arenas in which to find the self-esteem that was missing in his life. Gary had a variety of jobs until he became too weak to work—taxi driver, home remodeling, answering service, city maintenance department, deckhand, and flower delivery. In every setting Gary felt inferior. He longed for his employer and co-workers to tell him that he did good work, that his job was worthwhile, or that he looked good on the job.

Failing to be affirmed at home or at work, Gary turned to sex and drugs as means to feel good about himself. Hallucinogens and amphetamines were his drugs of choice. Anonymous and multiple partners became an acceptable substitute for the long-term relationship that he desired. Gary would go out once or twice a week, accepting whatever sexual offers came his way. He concluded that there is "nothing good in life other than sex," since it was only at these times that he felt good about himself.

A man he met during one of these adventures became

his lover. Two years into the relationship he told his stepfather that he was gay. His stepfather took the disclosure as an opportunity to tell Gary how to live. His mother refused to talk about what Gary subsequently discovered she had thought since he was in high school. After four years the relationship with his lover ended. It took seven years, by Gary's count, for him to get over it. During these seven years Gary reverted back to his routine of anonymous and multiple sexual partners.

In April 1984 Gary noticed that his lymph glands were swollen. He went to a physician, who told him that he had ARC. The diagnosis surprised Gary. He knew that he was possibly infectious and surely vulnerable to infection. However, his sexual activities had become something of a compulsion. It was difficult for him to accept the fact that he carried a fatal venereal disease. It took him six months totally to stop engaging in sexual activity.

He had known four men who had been told that they had ARC or AIDS. They were all dying as far as he was concerned, even if they didn't want to admit it. The news regarding his own condition was an additional incentive for him to hurry and spend time with them. The uncertainties related to his own future worried him. He didn't know what was best for him to do, what treatment to seek, whom to tell, whether to continue working, or how to alter his social life. The answers to these questions would depend on whether he remained stable, progressed to an AIDS diagnosis, or could foresee his death. He genuinely felt that all he was doing and would do became pointless when he was diagnosed. However, like his view of his life, he decided to "pretend that it meant something, even though it didn't."

In August 1985 Gary developed a lung infection that changed his diagnosis from ARC to AIDS. His view of himself and the world changed once again. The future became more certain. He felt "horrible." Despite his low self-esteem, Gary believed that he had worked hard, that he had worked through a lot of problems. And even though he had no resources and felt that people often had taken advantage of him, he still felt that he had something to offer the world. But alas, all is lost. Gary feels that a good portion of his life has been wasted and that his long-term goals are hopelessly beyond reach.

Gary became too weak to work an eight-hour day. He found a part-time job, but it paid little. He told his parents that he had no place to go and that he had ARC. He misrepresented his diagnosis for several reasons. Their dream of middle-class respectability was falling apart because of financial reversals that were pushing them into bankruptcy. Also, the problems between himself and them had never been resolved fully. To tell them the truth, in his mind, would have meant losing them. They had been unable or unwilling to share his problems before. He felt certain that a disclosure of this magnitude would be too disruptive of their drive for an "ideal" family for them to accept.

His parents allowed him to return home, but he was asked to live in a garage room. His presence inside the house would have been too disruptive. Gary didn't care. He was happy to be separated from the arguing and fighting that was taking place between his parents. The less time that he was with them acting as a referee, the better he liked it.

Gary continued to work half-time during the three months that he lived in the garage. Even though he was getting weaker, after work he would go home, prepare dinner for the family, clean up the kitchen, and do other chores around the house. His parents were quite willing for him to do this. They were not willing, however, to risk using the same dishes that he did. His were marked with tape. Gary felt that this sort of treatment was consistent with their past efforts to take advantage of him. After all, his stepfather had him unknowingly sign papers years ago that resulted in Gary's being denied an inheritance from a grandparent. Why should he now, even if he told them the truth that he has AIDS, expect them to treat him more kindly. In Gary's words, "If I wasn't worthy of their love and respect before, I surely wouldn't deserve it now."

Gary moved from the garage room to a residence provided by a local AIDS support organization. He can reside there as long as he is able to take care of himself. At that point Gary will have no place to go except, in his words, "to the hospital to die." He is not able to work. He has talked with a lawyer about giving someone power of attorney to make decisions regarding his medical care if he becomes unable to do so. Unfortunately, there is no one he trusts enough to give power over his life. Everyone has either withdrawn or thrown him out. He thinks that his mother or stepfather would agree to be his surrogate, but he is afraid that they would let him die just to be rid of him.

Gary looks at his illness as he has looked at everything else that has happened to him: "AIDS is just one more 'slap in the face' to deal with." In retrospect, he regrets not separating from his family long ago. He was smart enough to realize that they were abusing him, but he was too passive to do anything about it. In his mind, all the abuse he took was his fault, not theirs. Gary does not regret, however, being gay. He wouldn't change this part of himself even if he could. He had one "wonderful love relationship" and several "good affairs." His homosexuality, like AIDS and so much else in his experience, is "a burden to be turned into an opportunity to learn and to grow."

It is perhaps paradoxical that with AIDS, Gary has

found the affirmation, attention, and acceptance (at least from a few people) that he always sought. The men and women who provide his medical care have become his family. The people who oversee and live in the facility where he resides treat him like a person whose life matters, not as if he no longer mattered. People are now doing things for him without expecting anything in return. For example, one volunteer asked him about his favorite food. "Smoked oysters" was his reply. The next day Gary found in the refrigerator smoked oysters with his name on them. Other people are giving him small amounts of money to supplement his $237 monthly Social Security income. These people, and the physicians and nurses who care for him, are, to him, "unselfish people who have come to me and shared what they were able in order to make my life better." At last and in extreme circumstances, Gary is at peace with himself. Dying doesn't bother him now. Of course, the physical losses are frightening to him. But he can do nothing about it. His life has been a mixture of joy and sorrow. So when death comes, Gary thinks that it will be a positive event. "I'll feel good about dying. Anyone should if they are at peace with themselves."

Gary's peace does not result from conforming his conduct to the mores of churches or from knowing and accepting orthodox religious doctrines. As might be expected from parents striving to be an ideal family, Gary was taken to Sunday school every week until he finished elementary school. The family continued to attend Sunday morning worship sevices until he was a sophomore in high school. During his junior year he began to break away from his parents and their expectations for him. As with his sexuality, Gary wanted to come to terms with his own religious beliefs. He wondered if he could find some reason to feel good about himself in religion. He wanted to discover if there was anything in religion that would validate his existence.

He has attended several churches—Methodist, Assembly of God, Roman Catholic, Baptist, Presbyterian, Metropolitan Community Church. In his own way Gary has come to conclude that there is a God: "Life can't be an accident. There must be a source. And God must be it." Further, Gary now thinks that life is good and each person is special in God's sight. As such, Gary reasons that one continues to exist even when one loses one's own body. This eternal life, according to Gary, is a state of being at one with God.

When he was younger, Gary was troubled about God's judgment of homosexuality. This no longer is a source of concern. He reasons: "Even if I'm doing wrong, God will forgive me. God surely wants us to be who we are, to be honest with and about ourselves. If we make mistakes, we may have to pay for them. But at the time we make them, we did what we could, what was important at that time. I've had sex with countless men who said they were married and had children. I'm no better or worse than they are. If they are OK with God, so am I. After all, God made me. I'm gay. It must be OK."

Gary's existence was not validated in the churches. It seems, however, that it has been validated as a result of his quest to make sense of himself, life, and AIDS. The diagnosis of AIDS caused him to wrestle more earnestly with these issues: "I've been enlightened. But, unfortunately, it's a terminal disease."

Gary thinks that churches have little desire to help people with AIDS. They seem to do what they can in order not to change their negative views of homosexuality or to redefine their responsibilities to people with AIDS. Gary refuses to judge or condemn the people in the pews. He believes that churchgoers need to think they're better than other people. Gary is critical, however, of church leaders who won't lead people in overcoming their hypocrisy. In short, Gary is not bitter toward the church or those who attend. As far as he is concerned, "life is a good thing. No need to be negative now. AIDS isn't God's punishment on me or anyone else. The virus has no sense. It doesn't know what it's doing. A lot in the world is not fair. It's an imperfect world. I can accept what is. Oh, I hate to go when I feel like I want so much to be here for other people. If I followed certain religious rules, maybe I would have lived longer. So maybe I've brought this on myself. But I'm not the sort of person who is able to conform. I just had to work with who I am and what I had. I feel blessed. I've lived thirty-six years. That is a long time when compared to the twenty- and twenty-one-year-old guys who have AIDS. Some of them have not come to terms with life and God. I have. As I said before, I think that death will be positive for me. When it comes, I'm ready. Anyone would be if they are at peace with themselves."

RICHARD

Richard was an artist. He loved colors, textures, and shapes. After being graduated with a degree in art, Richard worked for a small firm as a graphics artist. He enjoyed working on one project and then another. The variety of assignments allowed him to experiment with his innate talent and test his training. Richard was a perfectionist. No project was acceptable until he was satisfied that he had done the best he could. The excitement and challenge of creating something attractive made getting out of bed every morning a special pleasure.

Richard migrated to Texas from New Jersey when he was twenty-six years old. His father, twin sister, and older brother continued to live in New Jersey. His mother died when he was twenty-three. After her death Richard stopped dating women, accepted his homosexuality, and began dating men. He was old-fashioned. He never participated in anonymous sex acts. He preferred to meet a person, get to know him, and spend time together. By the time Richard became ill, he had "slept with" approximately twenty-five men over a period of four years.

Richard told his father that he was gay before he moved to Houston. His father said little at that time. Richard's sexuality was never discussed by them again, even though Richard visited him about once every other year and spoke by phone about four times a year. Richard's twin was more acceptant of him. She visited him and his lover shortly before he became ill. The three of them had a good visit together. She was shown the sights in Houston, and seemingly she felt at ease eating out with them and going to a gay dance bar. Richard and his older brother had never been close. Richard was imaginative and creative. His brother was an ex-marine who worked in a factory. Their relationship became even more distant and formal after Richard told him about himself. Regardless of his family's response, Richard felt good about being gay. He liked to look good. His hair was always groomed. He maintained his weight at 160 pounds. His clothing fit nicely on his 5½-foot frame. In short, Richard was proud to be a man and especially proud to be a gay man. This pride in himself was responsible for his break with the Roman Catholic Church. Richard felt that it was hypocritical to participate in a church that condemned him for who he was.

Richard met Charles in May 1981. Richard was almost twenty-eight; Charles was twenty-two, recently graduated from college, and new to Houston. They became lovers later that year. A small condo was purchased. Plans were made for the future. They pursued their careers. Neither of them used drugs. They drank little alcohol. They were both raised in the Roman Catholic Church but almost never attended mass. They characterized themselves as "the happy little gay couple working to have their cottage with a white picket fence around the yard." Their friends were mostly heterosexual couples and single men or women. AIDS was something happening to other gay men, not them. They felt a bit smug about it all. They simply didn't fit the profile of the men who got AIDS. Their illusion of invulnerability began to shatter in August 1982.

At first Richard attributed his fatigue, shortness of breath, fever, and persistent cough to a recurrent cold or the flu. He put off going to a physician. The small firm for which he worked didn't provide medical insurance coverage for its employees. Richard purchased a private policy but understood that coverage would not begin until it had been in force for one year. By April 1983 Richard could not ignore his condition any longer. He was diagnosed with *Pneumocystis carinii* pneumonia. Because he didn't have hospitalization insurance, Charles paid his hospital bill and for his home treatment. AIDS, the disease that Richard and Charles thought happened to other people, thus became a central feature of their lives and relationship.

Richard returned to work after three weeks of treatment and rest. He told the man and woman who owned the firm that he had AIDS. The woman ran from the room crying. She was shocked, grief-stricken, and afraid that Richard was a threat to her health. He was moved to a private work space. But after Richard's physician spoke with his employers, he was moved back to his former work space that was shared by three other designers. From this time until Richard had to quit work, in March 1985, he was treated with respect and compassion at work.

Richard was angry at first about having AIDS. He felt that the media sensationalized the disease. The way the disease and the people with it were portrayed by the media was exploitative, in his judgment. He thought that the distortions regarding the risks of infection were being used by homophobic people to justify discrimination against gay men, whether or not they were ill. Had AIDS first appeared in heterosexual, Republican, white bankers, Richard was certain that the media would have designed their coverage to evoke a sympathetic rather than a fearful public response.

Between April 1983 and June 1985 Richard had recurrent pneumonias and fungal infections that required hospitalization. His medical care was being provided in a state institution. That he didn't have insurance or savings became irrelevant. Although he was grateful for the quality and character of care that he received in the hospital and at the clinic, he disliked the"Flash Gordon" costumes (masks, gowns, and gloves) that people had to wear when entering his hospital room. In an effort to poke fun at what Richard found objectionable, Charles took a life-sized cardboard cutout of Joan Collins, used to promote her autobiography, to the hospital. (Richard enjoyed her role in the television series *Dynasty*.) Before taking the prop into Richard's room, Charles draped it with a mask and gown. Richard loved it. So did the nurses and orderlies. The physicians never seemed to understand the joke.

Richard gradually worked through his anger about having AIDS. He wanted to go on living, loving, and working. He conscientiously took prophylactic drugs, ate a balanced diet, and rested as much as possible. Richard tended to stay away from the clinic. No one is quite sure why he was reluctant to ask for medical help. It seemed to Charles that Richard felt that going to his physician was a reminder that he was no longer the robust, healthy, weight-lifting, gay ideal.

When Richard was initially diagnosed and while he was receiving IV drugs at home, he called his father to tell him about his illness. Richard's father said little. A note from him arrived in the mail. The message was short: "Words are difficult in a time like this. Just remember that I love you." Despite this putatively supportive message, Richard's father did not tell Richard's sister and brother that Richard had AIDS, which Richard had asked him to do. Richard phoned them both after a few days. His only comment was "they don't understand." He thought that his family wanted to ignore it all, hoping that the illness or his probable death would just go away.

His illness did not go away. Family and friends did, however. His already small circle of friends became smaller as time passed and his overall condition deteriorated. This was due in part to the desertion by some of his friends and in part to Richard's withdrawal. He remarked, "I don't have time or energy to deal with friends or issues that don't mean anything to me. I'd rather concentrate on those three or four people who do mean something to me and let the rest go."

Richard's family basically deserted him during his illness. No one visited. Flowers never arrived when he was in the hospital. Supportive phone calls were few and far between. Nevertheless, Richard tried to stay in touch with his family, especially his twin sister. She was to marry in February 1985. Richard wanted very much to attend the wedding. By then his weight had dropped to 100 pounds. He saved enough money for the round trip air fare to New Jersey. His best suit was altered to fit him better. New shoes were purchased. His father and sister gave him permission to attend the wedding. Richard was planning to stay at his father's house.

The evening of his arrival was a disaster. His sister told him not to tell her fiancé that he was gay or that he had AIDS. Richard was hurt and angrily responded: "What the hell do you think I planned to do? Do you think that I planned to wear a sandwich board with 'I'm queer' on one side and 'I have AIDS' on the other while I parade up and down the church aisles?" Richard stayed at home one night, returning to Houston the next day without seeing his twin marry. He said, "I felt like a leper. No one wanted to touch me. My brother wouldn't bring his wife or child into the house. They kept asking me how I felt but never seemed to hear anything that I said. If I coughed, they pulled away." Richard never saw any of his family again. His sister sent him pictures of the wedding. Richard returned them unopened: "What do I want with pictures of a wedding where I wasn't welcomed?"

One month later Richard had to quit work. His weakness and frequent trips to the clinic made it impossible for him to continue. Only then did Richard believe that AIDS would kill him. He began to talk to Charles about his death. He worried about how Charles would manage the house when he was "gone." Richard knew that Charles was a klutz around the house. Unfinished household projects consumed his time and energy. Richard frequently told Charles, "Be nice to George. George can take care of you after I'm gone." George, a heterosexual friend, was good with tools and liked to work on household projects.

Richard also began to talk more about his mother and how badly she had been treated by his family. Often he would draw parallels between how she was treated and how he was being treated. She was put into a nursing home and left to die. Richard said to Charles, "She was a good, loving woman who never hurt a soul. They treated her like a dog after she became ill. Since we've been treated alike by the family, it would be fitting if we were buried together. After I'm cremated, try to bury my ashes next to her." Richard began to cry. These were the first tears Charles saw Richard shed.

During July 1985 Richard started on another experimental drug. The side effects made him so uncomfortable that the drug was stopped after two weeks. He told the nurse, "All I have left in life is the two dollars in my back pocket and my dignity. The time I have left I want to be quality time, not time eaten up by a drug that only makes me sick." Within two weeks Richard was back in the clinic complaining of headaches and trouble with his vision. He was found to have CMV (cytomegalovirus) retinitis, a viral infection of the eye that can lead to blindness. There is no standard therapy for infections with this virus. One of the investigational drugs that has been somewhat efficacious was begun. Unfortunately, Richard had one strokelike and one psychotic reaction to the drug. The drug was stopped. Richard regained his mental function. His eyesight, however, worsened.

At about the same time Richard began to have neurological symptoms. He had trouble with his memory and coordination. Getting around the house became problematic. He could no longer cook for himself. His increasing dependency was stripping him of his dignity that he prized so highly. Richard felt that each new loss "didn't matter." When he was asked if he wanted to try another drug, he responded, "Don't bother." It was clear to the clinic personnel that as Richard's eyesight, motor, and memory problems worsened, his desire and will to live lessened.

Richard went home to die. He talked to Charles about his desire to stop taking his medicine. They knew that this action would hasten Richard's death. Richard gave

Charles power of attorney and prepared his will. Within weeks he was blind, too weak to get out of bed, had diarrhea, and was incontinent. Richard had decided that life no longer had the quality to make it worth living. He wanted to die at home, without tubes in his arms, and with Charles at his side. All this was extremely difficult for Charles, who now was twenty-six. His part of the story is told in the next chapter.

It took Richard four weeks to die. He lay in his lightless world wasting away. He had his thirtieth birthday during the second week of his dying. Charles read birthday cards to him. A neighbor baked him a cake that he couldn't see. Charles fed him part of a piece of his birthday cake and held a glass of champagne from which he sipped. Richard asked to talk to his twin sister. In tears, he told her that he wanted to see her before he died. She couldn't continue the conversation. Later that day she called and spoke with Charles. He repeated Richard's request, but she made no commitments.

After Richard's birthday he refused every offer of solid or liquid nourishment. He sipped water. A priest administered the sacrament of the sick. Hospice personnel visited every few days to monitor his condition. Charles hired a licensed visiting nurse to help with Richard's care four hours a day. Gradually his frail, eighty-pound body drew into a fetal position. He looked more and more like the countless people who died in wartime concentration camps. At a time when no one other than Charles was in the house, an eerie sound came from Richard's bedroom. Charles rushed to the room. Richard was gasping for breath. Charles held his hand, stroked his head, wept, and told Richard that he loved him, that he was there. Then Richard breathed no more. This brave young man who valued his dignity and privacy seemed somehow to have known that this was the first time in days that he and Charles were alone. He had wanted his death to be a private event for him and Charles. And so it was.

Charles called Richard's sister to tell her that Richard had died. She was told of Richard's request for his cremated remains to be buried with or next to his mother. Charles was told that the family had decided already not to be responsible for Richard's funeral or preparation of his body for burial. She said that she would discuss Richard's wish for burial with her family and call Charles when a decision was reached. Seven days later she called to tell Charles that they didn't want Richard's ashes. The family that was distant from Richard in life and absent during his bout with a terminal illness remained consistent. They rejected him even in death.

BOB

Bob, a sensitive, intelligent, young man, wanted to be a physician. After being graduated from college with a degree in biology, he was accepted for admission by two medical schools. Registration was delayed because Bob needed to work and save money in order to pay his way. He taught biology at his alma mater for one year. Then he began working for a major electronics firm in Texas. His commitment to set aside money for medical school waned as his work began to be transformed into a career. The delayed gratification associated with a career in medicine became less attractive as his income and career advanced rapidly in the electronics firm. The job that initially was intended to be a short-term commitment turned into an eight-year occupation.

A managerial position in a telecommunications firm

was Bob's next step on the career ladder. His work was evaluated highly. Promotions and salary increases were regular features of his five years of service. When he left the firm in 1981 to move to Houston to work in real estate sales and investment, his salary was more than $45,000 per year plus fringes. Houston's real estate market turned sour in 1983. This decline coincided with the onset of his symptoms of ARC.

Bob married while he was working at the electronics firm. The birth of a daughter expanded the family to three. Bob's parents were proud of their only child, his family, and his advancing career. Despite their pleasure and Bob's effort to conform to a heterosexual life-style, Bob could not honestly suppress any longer the homosexual feelings that he had had since puberty. He divorced his wife, left the Baptist church in which he had been active, left the electronics firm for a job with the telecommunications firm, and began to claim his homosexual identity. He never told his wife or daughter that he is gay and ill. His daughter is with her mother. Bob sees her twice a year.

Bob's entry into gay life came only after the divorce from his wife. He never was intimate with a man until then. Even though he was thirty years old when he came out, Bob was not in a hurry to experience every facet of gay life. He preferred having a small group of friends with whom he could build lasting relationships. Also, he preferred to date rather than to have many tricks. The values that he embraced before coming out were carried into his homosexual life-style. He is a man of moderation, integrity, goals, and ability. He felt good about his decision to be true to himself when it was made and continues to do so.

Life as a single, gay man was exciting for Bob. The ballet, galleries, museums, symphony, and restaurants regularly were part of his social life with a small group of close friends. Trips to a gay bar also were part of their life together, but they were a minor part compared with his other interests, which include photography, travel, tennis, and piano. His life-style began to change in the spring of 1983, around the date of his thirty-fifth birthday.

Severe itching was the first physical symptom that something was wrong. His physician prescribed Valium. It brought him little relief. Then he periodically would have night sweats, brief episodes of diarrhea, mild headaches, and fatigue. By winter Bob was diagnosed with chronic hepatitis. Working a full day became less possible as the seasons changed from spring to winter. He did part-time sales work for a while. But by the start of 1984 Bob simply did not have the stamina to take care of himself and to work on a regular schedule. Now he works at odd jobs when he is able. He began to worry that his several physical problems were indicative of AIDS. He was relieved to discover that he "only has ARC." However, he knew that the less severe diagnosis was no guarantee that he would survive or that he will not ultimately progress to AIDS.

Bob has put his education in biology to work. He goes to a medical library every few weeks to read recently published articles about the AIDS virus, the disease, and its complications. He has known four persons who had AIDS. All of them have been diagnosed since he became ill. Three of them have died. Only one of the four was a "fast-laner." The oldest member of this quartet was fifty-five, and the others a few years younger than Bob. As each one has died and as the fourth continues to deteriorate, Bob wonders what will happen to himself. All of death associated with AIDS seems to be "such a waste" to him. He grieves the deaths of friends, not only his loss of them, but also their loss of themselves.

One death in particular was hard for Bob, a black man, to accept. Barry was a "beautiful white man who modeled for gay magazines that are comparable to *Playboy* or *Hustler*. Barry never told anyone that he was ill. He was too proud for that. His loss of weight signaled us that something was wrong." Bob and Barry were close friends. Bob asked his roommate, who is an excellent watercolor artist, to paint Barry's portrait from a picture made when Barry was well. The portrait was finished three days before Barry died. Bob gave the portrait to Barry's lover, who displayed it at Barry's memorial service.

These deaths and the uncertainty about his infectivity depresses Bob at times. His sadness stems from a more or less self-imposed isolation. Bob would like to be a boyfriend again to a man he dated previously. He hesitates to make his interests known. Even if the man responded positively, Bob doubts that he could act on his desire because of his concern not to infect anyone. As an acceptable compromise, Bob sees him at least once a week. But Bob's needs for touching and intimacy are not being met. In Bob's words, "I'm way behind on my quota of hugs." Bob stopped being sexually active when he was told that he has ARC.

Bob feels close to his mother and father, who are both retired. Although they live in another city, he sees them every four months. They either visit each other or meet to play in card tournaments. Bob told them that he is gay and that he is ill. Their response to his first disclosure consisted of two questions. "Is this why you got divorced?" "Are you happier now?" Bob answered yes to both questions. Their summary response was, "Fine, your happiness is what is important." His second disclosure was purposely veiled. He does not want to alarm them. They were told that he does not have AIDS, which is true. Bob indicated that he might be infected with the AIDS virus, so that they should not be totally surprised if his condition worsens. Their response to his second disclosure was as affirming as their first response. They promised to help in any way that they could. Bob was invited to return home if he wished, an offer he has refused at present. Their relationship has not been affected by either revelation. They continue to speak by phone once or twice weekly.

Apart from his parents, Bob has told no one that he has ARC. He isn't afraid of being rejected. In his mind it simply is no one's business as long as he doesn't represent a threat to anyone's health. Bob believes that his roommate suspects that he has ARC, even though they have not discussed it. Bob views his condition as a private matter. It has provided him with time and an incentive to gain more insight into himself. He has learned how to appreciate the little things in life that are too frequently overlooked, depreciated, or ignored, and at the age of forty, life's intricacies have taken on a new significance for him. Life, all forms of life, have become objects of wonder. Despite his education in biology, the processes of life have taken on a new. significance now that the immune function in his body is disordered. Observation and reflection have become ways not only to pass time, but also to appreciate and better understand how awe-inspiring and precious life is.

Each day has become a blessing for Bob. It provides an opportunity to enjoy people, to understand their differences and similarities, and to discover their good qualities. Bob says, "Everyone begins with one hundred points now." This presumption reflects Bob's constitutional emotional attraction to people. He presumes that a person has integrity and is worthy of his friendship until he is proven wrong. He longs for relationships but believes that his diagnosis and preoccupation with it stop him from establishing emotional ties that he or another person may not be able to sustain.

Bob has become more introspective since he has been ill. He considered once that AIDS was God's retribution on homosexuals. He entertained this notion for "maybe thirty seconds" before he considered it foolishness. After leaving the Baptist church when he divorced his wife and claimed his homosexuality, he attended Catholic mass weekly for about eight years. He has not been related to a congregation or attended worship during the past two years. This absence from church, however, doesn't mean that his interest in God has lapsed. On the contrary, Bob has given more thought than ever to God's relationship with humanity and the nature of moral conduct.

The doctrines of the Christian church are not fully understood. He hasn't figured out the relationship of God to Jesus, what all this means, or its significance. If he better understood doctrines, perhaps he would be able to use that knowledge to become a better person and be able to relate better to other people. He has tried to live by the Golden Rule. If he conducts himself according to it, then he feels he meets the test of morality. At times he doubts that God accepts homosexuality. But then he considers this proposition more fully. "Homosexuality," for Bob, "is not what one does sexually. It is an emotional desire. It's still love. Everything that can exist in heterosexual relationships can exist in homosexual relationships. If God approves of one, then God must approve of the other. The quality of the emotional commitment is what is important, not the gender of the parties. AIDS is no indication of God's view of homosexuality. God didn't send AIDS, chicken pox, or smallpox on any particular person or group of people. If it rains, some people will get wet. It's as simple as that."

Bob prays every day. Mostly he prays for the well-being of others. He doesn't believe that the whole world revolves around him. He would like to be freed of the AIDS virus. But in his words, "if eighty to ninety percent of all people with AIDS could be cured, and not me, then I'd go with the eighty to ninety percent." The church, according to Bob, could help people with AIDS if it would. Bob would like to see the church educate people about AIDS, shape public opinion, help families to deal with their stress, and help patients to cope with disease and death. Again, in Bob's words, "Falwell says something stupid about AIDS or gay people and it gets front-page coverage. Someone else says something sensible or does something charitable and the media ignore it."

Bob's message to the church and to the public is "to quit panicking. The AIDS virus isn't *that* contagious. Direct all this nervous energy into helping people who have been infected and those institutions trying to find a cure. Stop running scared, closing doors. Now is the time not to close doors on people. Open them. Hug the people in more than a physical sense. The huggees need it and deserve it. And the huggers will learn something about what it means to be human in the process."

ALAN

Alan describes himself as "high screech." He is gregarious, energetic, and compulsive. Opera, ballet, and theater interest him. Fast and easy sex in "costume baths," where he could act out his sexual fantasies, also was an interest.

Like Gary earlier, Alan was intended to be the perfect only child in a perfect home. And, like Bob, dating women and planning for marriage were seen to be the sort of thing that a man does naturally. But marriage and perfection, as determined by someone else, were not natural to Alan. He discovered that he could not and would not be what he isn't.

After finishing college Alan returned home to work in his family's business. He dated a woman, grew to love her, had intercourse once, and planned a marriage. No one knew, however, that from age thirteen until he went away to college, Alan was having sex with a workman in the family business' warehouse. Alan had told his parents that he felt ambivalent about his sexuality. He asked them to let him see a psychiatrist. They didn't see the need for this. After all, with the impending marriage, the questions or suspicions of friends, church people, and business associates regarding Alan's sexuality would be put to rest. Final arrangements were made as the wedding date approached. His fiancée's wedding dress had been purchased. The reception had been planned in every detail. But as the wedding day neared, Alan felt that he could not live a charade. He could not bring himself to deceive his fiancée any longer. He knew that he had to try one more time to tell his parents that he is gay.

Even before Alan met his future fiancée he decided that he was not truly ambivalent about his sexuality. He was gay. He knew it. He wanted his parents to know it, but they seemed unwilling or unable to let him tell them the truth about himself. Alan lived a double life. He maintained a heterosexual image for the benefit of his parents and their peers. He engaged in homosexual conduct for his own benefit. The compromise that he thought would be acceptable failed. In a desperate attempt to let his parents know the truth about him before the planned wedding occurred, Alan took his parents to see *Making Love*, a movie about a married young man who feels drawn to gay meeting places and who subsequently affirms his homosexuality.

On returning home Alan read a "treatise" to them in which he emphatically proclaimed to them, and the world, that he is gay. His handwritten, twelve-page message tells them, in short, that he loves them unconditionally and forever, that he appreciates all they have done for him, that for unknown reasons he has always been attracted to men, that he is gay and does not wish to change, that he likes and feels good about himself, that they must be hurt but his sexuality is not their fault, that being honest with them is a source of personal happiness, that he wants them to respect him even if they don't approve of his sexual conduct, and that he is willing to do what he can to help them understand him. A furious argument followed. Alan struck his father. He accused his mother of being a "latent lesbian." As might be expected, the marriage was canceled.

As Alan entered gay life he felt like a kid in a candy shop. He went to bars seven nights a week. He had no role models. He thought that this was what gay men did. Sex was reinterpreted for him. Before coming out he thought intercourse was a special, consummating act. But with his plunge into that part of gay life where sexual contact was an end in itself, Alan set his more "provincial" views about sex aside. He gravitated to establishments where anonymous contacts were readily available. Conversation, credentials, or character were not important in these settings. They provided an ideal environment for Alan, who confesses to having low self-esteem. Here he could comfortably act out his sexual fantasies. He could experience what he let pass for "intimacy" with another man. Taking a man to his home was impossible. There were reminders of Mom, Dad, and God at home. Under no circumstances could he experience the same freedom there that he felt in alternate settings.

Alan's sexual conduct took its toll on his body. He has been treated for many sexually transmitted diseases. He has chronic hepatitis and chronic genital herpes. His immune system is impaired. In short, Alan was diagnosed with ARC in 1983. He has modified his life-style in light of his condition. Now he is sexually abstinent. The death of his best friend from AIDS shortly after he was diagnosed with ARC helped him to make this decision. The deaths of other men that he knew has helped him to maintain his resolve. Now he is quite obsessive about his health. "Alan the libertine" has become "Alan the nun."

In retrospect, Alan regrets that his self-esteem was so low that he felt his only avenue of affirmation was in settings conducive to dangerous conduct. If his home and societal environment had been more acceptant of homosexuality, perhaps, Alan reasons, what he and others have risked would not have been felt necessary. In an accepting environment perhaps he would not have terminated the few "relationships" that he had after a few months. He thinks that society in general is both overtly and subtly hostile to homosexual people, conduct, and relationships. AIDS, in his view, is an excuse for society to isolate and oppress people that are disliked anyway. In Alan's words, "calling discrimination public health doesn't make it right."

Alan told his parents that he is immunocompromised. They are aware of his hepatitis and herpes. He has not told them about his infection with the AIDS virus. He thinks that this is all they really want to know. Alan's father still denies that Alan is gay. He prays to God that it just isn't so. His mother believes that Alan is gay. Even so, she wishes that he would marry, have a child, and maintain a gay relationship on the side. Alan is not permitted to speak of his gay friends to his parents or have them in his parents' home. He feels so unaccepted in his parents' home that he spent less than a total of one hour with them on Thanksgiving and Christmas Day last year.

He is fatalistic about his disease. Alan expects to die earlier than he would have because of his past behavior. He is confident that he'll progress to AIDS and then die. He has begun to dispose of some of his possessions in order to lessen his parents' burden of dealing with his affairs. His papers are being organized. He's cutting back on some of his activities and commitments. All this is being done because of what he sees as his probable future. He feels that he is being liberated as he reorders his life. Time has become his most precious possession. Living and enjoying quality relationships are now his top priorities. He feels that he is responsible for every twenty-four hours. He must choose well. Having come to these conclusions, Alan feels freer now than ever. He is determined to be himself. He has no time to "waste" conforming his life to the expectations of others. He wants to absorb fully each experience and then move on to new experiences. Being in control of his life has become important. Having been a member of Alcoholics Anonymous and Sex Addicts Anonymous, Alan is "fully aware of how little power people can have over their lives." Any form of dependency is fearful to him now, including the sort of physical dependencies that some people with AIDS develop. Rather than being in that state, Alan thinks that suicide is a valid option. Suicide, for him, is not a choice to be made lightly. Nevertheless, it is a way to have control over oneself, even as one dies.

Part of Alan's low self-esteem results from being told in his church that homosexual people are sinners and homosexual conduct is sinful. When he became an adult he stopped participating in his home, tall-steeple church. He has rejected his church, but he has not rejected God. He feels sorry for the several clergy that he knows are gay. Their ministerial gifts have been affirmed by prestigious appointments. Nevertheless, Alan laments that they have had to live a lie in order to pursue their calling. The church should grow up, Alan thinks. Sticking its head in the sand and leaving it there, hoping that homosexuality and AIDS will disappear, won't make this happen. Alan thinks the notion that AIDS is punishment from God is "hogwash." The God that Alan knows doesn't act this way. Alan's God is all-loving. Traditional dogmas and doctrines are irrelevant to spirituality. Religiosity, according to him, is meaningless. How a person loves in response to God's love is what is important. God doesn't send people problems, only opportunities. People can respond positively or negatively. By so doing, people make life heaven or hell.

For Alan, at thirty years of age, ARC has been an opportunity to reorder his life, to sort out priorities, to learn honesty and courage, to value time, people, and loving relationships, and to be liberated from the judgments of institutions and people that he is unworthy of love.

BRYAN

Bryan was twenty-four when he was diagnosed with ARC in January 1985. Three months later he was hospitalized with *P. carinii* pneumonia and diagnosed as having AIDS. When Bryan was first seen by the authors in August 1985, he commented that he was "scared to death." Reasons for his fear became known as months of contact with Bryan passed.

Bryan told his parents in 1980 that he is gay. His

father's response was "surprisingly supportive." His mother felt hurt. She cried. As days passed after his disclosure, Bryan's relationship with his mother deteriorated. Bryan's brother, who is three years older, and sister, who is two years younger, were also told of his homosexuality. His sister's response indicated that the disclosure was a "non-event," it just didn't matter to her. Bryan's brother, however, was overtly hostile. The brothers argued and physically fought. These battles would erupt when Bryan's brother was drinking alcohol. Bryan describes both his brother and mother as alcoholics. He decided that it would be better for him if he moved out on his own.

Bryan went to Texas to go to school. His father paid his tuition and living expenses. They were an upper-middle-class family. Bryan lived well, dressed expensively, and was given four new cars between his sixteenth and twenty-second birthdays. Each new car replaced a previous new car that had been wrecked. Life went blissfully for Bryan, despite the alienation from his mother and brother, until 1982, when his father died. His father's considerable estate went to his mother. She closed the family purse to Bryan. He began to work full time during the summer and part time during the remainder of the year to meet his school and living expenses.

Four months after his father's death his mother died, early in 1983. Her estate was left to Bryan's older brother. Bryan and his sister received nothing—Bryan because he is gay, his sister because of her mother's disapproval of her fiancé, who was "beneath their station." By this time Bryan's brother had moved to the same city in Texas where Bryan goes to school. Friends began to tell Bryan in October 1983 that his brother was seen in some of the local gay bars. Finally, Bryan encountered his brother in a bar. His brother admitted being gay and said that he had decided to keep his sexuality secret, since their mother reacted so negatively to Bryan's disclosure. Now that she had died, Bryan's brother felt free to come out of the closet. Even though both brothers now knew of their common sexuality, the relationship between them did not improve. Bryan received no financial assistance from his brother. Neither did his sister.

Bryan's routine of work and school was interrupted two or three times a week to go out with his gay friends. About three times a month he would meet someone "interesting" who would be a sex partner. One sex partner became his lover. They had lived together for fourteen months when the relationship ended in December 1984. Unhappy about the failed relationship and the stresses he felt trying to balance school, work, and home, Bryan decided to start a new year and a new life in Kentucky, where an uncle and paternal grandparents live. He planned to live with his grandparents until he could have his own place. He ended up staying with his uncle, however, because his grandparents were ill and barely able to sustain themselves on their income from social security.

Bryan's uncle is married and has an eight-year-old son. The second week in his uncle's home Bryan noticed white patches in his mouth. Also, he got the flu. His uncle suspected that Bryan is gay. When asked, Bryan confirmed his uncle's suspicions. His uncle told his son to stay away from Bryan. He also told Bryan to leave the house, even though he had no money and no place to go. A physician at the public hospital who was treating Bryan came to his rescue. Bryan was admitted to the hospital. Further testing indicated that he had ARC. The hospital agreed to pay Bryan's fare back to the city in Texas where he went to school. His uncle, who was told the diagnosis, gathered Bryan's belongings and took him to the bus station after he was discharged from the hospital. Before releasing Bryan's belongings to him, he required Bryan to sign an IOU for approximately $200, the cost his uncle estimated for his room and board while Bryan was in his home. Bryan's uncle told him, "The only time I want to hear from you is when you pay your bill."

Bryan returned to work when he arrived in Texas. He continued to develop more symptoms of immune compromise—diarrhea, fatigue, weight loss, and finally, shortness of breath. In April 1985 he was hospitalized for *P. carinii* pneumonia. His diagnosis changed from ARC to AIDS. He was depressed, angry, and afraid. He began to dream about dying. He would awaken drenched in sweat and terrified. Bryan called his brother and told him what was happening. His brother visited but didn't offer to help. Bryan called his sister to tell her his diagnosis. By now she had married, has three preschool children, and lives in a distant state. She was concerned but, unlike Bryan's brother, was in no position to offer more than emotional support. Bryan was successfully treated for his pneumonia, but he was too weak to work after being released from the hospital. He couldn't pay rent so he was evicted from his apartment. From then until now, Bryan has either lived with a friend or gathered enough money to rent a room for a time.

Bryan was referred to Houston for followup care. Since being seen initially in August 1985, Bryan has made weekly bus trips to Houston to participate in medical experiments to stimulate his immune system. He arrives the night before his clinic appointment. Another patient with AIDS who felt sorry for Bryan picks him up at the bus station, lets him sleep on his sofa, and provides transportation to the bus for Bryan's return trip home.

As might be expected, Bryan feels alone, isolated,

afraid, and, at times, discouraged. He sees other patients in the clinic week to week. Their decline, which at times can be dramatic in its speed and severity, alarms Bryan. He wonders what his future will be. He worries about being sick and alone, except for a few old friends who have remained loyal and a few new friends he has made through the AIDS support organizations in his home city. Bryan tries to be optimistic, but it is difficult for him to adjust to being sick, dependent, alone, and destitute. His current situation contrasts starkly with his carefree excesses while his father was alive.

The most important project in Bryan's life now is to be reconciled with his family, especially his brother. Bryan admits that he abused many opportunities. So, in a sense, he feels that he really doesn't deserve to be helped financially. Nevertheless, Bryan loves his brother and would like to have his emotional support and become closer. They now talk but the conversations seem not to go anywhere. His brother gets drunk soon after finishing work each day. Thus, it is hard for Bryan to discern how his brother feels about him and the prospect of his death. Bryan's brother seems to delight in reminding Bryan about his sexual and financial irresponsibilities. Nevertheless, he tells Bryan that he doesn't want him to die. If he dies, however, he will be sure to give Bryan a nice funeral. Beyond this, Bryan should expect no help from him.

Bryan recognizes that the reconciliation with his brother that he seeks may never occur. He keeps trying but it seems to be a lost cause. Like his sister, Bryan's brother seems to want to avoid any conversation about the seriousness of Bryan's condition, a fact that Bryan is unable to forget physically or emotionally. His weakness and fear remind him of how vulnerable he is to infection and death. Bryan has learned from other people with AIDS what might happen to him. The potential suffering scares him more than the process of dying. He is adjusting to the latter prospect but is terrified by the former.

AIDS has revolutionized Bryan's life. Intimacy with his siblings has become more important. Similarly, intimacy, not necessarily sexual, with another man is a need once again. Finally, his faith in God and confidence in God's people has been affirmed. Bryan is a member of a Protestant denomination that does not condemn homosexual people or homosexual contact. He has no doubt that God loves him. AIDS is not God's punishment on him. As far as Bryan is concerned, he has AIDS because he was unlucky. God, in his mind, accepts him as he is—gay. Bryan is certain that God provides for his current needs. His faith in God and God's love for him, in Bryan's words, "will allow me to die a peaceful and serene death, soon if no cure for AIDS is found, or at a more distant time if there is a cure."

The pastor of the congregation where Bryan worships knows that he has AIDS. They talk frequently. A few people in the congregation are aware that he is ill. They treat him now as they did before. Their affirmation and courage not to withdraw have given Bryan strength to continue participating in worship services when he can. These sorts of pastoral and emotional supports are vital to Bryan's hope. These evidences of their concern for him have been reinforced by periodic monetary gifts from the congregation's benevolence fund. Unlike many people with AIDS, Bryan believes that he has not been abandoned by God or the church. These loyalties have enabled Bryan to retain some hope and sense of security. His spiritual family has helped to fill the void left by the withdrawal of his natural family.

KEVIN

AIDS is a personal and gay cultural experience for Kevin. The "cloud" hanging over gay men and other people about whom Kevin had been writing became his own in January 1985. An ominous purple spot appeared on his arm. Having known about AIDS since it was described in 1981, Kevin suspected the spot to be Kaposi's sarcoma. He was afraid. And as more lesions slowly have appeared on his skin, his worries about his health and future have grown.

Kevin, thirty-six, is reflective, educated, and articulate. He holds a bachelor degree in journalism and a master's degree in counseling. Further, he completed half the requirements for a doctorate in counseling and psychology. All his higher education has been at a prestigious northeastern university. He accepted his homosexuality in his early twenties, while at university. His talent as a writer and his interest in gay issues earned him the respect of publishers of predominantly gay-audience magazines and newspapers across the nation. As a result, Kevin has an extensive national network of politically active and issue-sensitive friends. Kevin tends to interpret AIDS in existential and sociopolitical terms.

Kevin is angry about AIDS. He is angry that he has it. His anger is a complex mixture of grief over a lost future, impatience with interruptions related to his medical care, frustration about contradictory medical opinions regarding treatment, and anxiety about not knowing what will happen to him next. At times his anger subsides. At other times it erupts, and he expresses it by pounding his fists on a wall or table in his apartment. In more reflective moments Kevin concludes: "Having AIDS is bad luck. Whatever the ingredients are that make certain people vulnerable to the virus, I happen to have them."

His mother and father have known about Kevin's sexuality for years. His father seems more able than his mother to accept Kevin the way he is. They were told that Kevin has AIDS. His mother's response is indicative

71

of how difficult it is for her to accept that Kevin is gay. Two comments reflect her ambivalence: "I thought only homosexuals got that." "You mean they let you walk around the streets with it?" She avoids the subject of AIDS in conversations with Kevin. She asks how he feels, but he senses that she really doesn't want to hear a detailed reply. Kevin thinks that her frequent assurance, "I think you'll be OK," comes because that is the way she wants it. A recovery would help her to deny the "awful truth" that she seems unable to hear.

Kevin's father seems better able to deal with Kevin's illness. He has responded to the fact of Kevin's illness in ways that convey a genuine concern. Despite what Kevin takes to be his evident concern, he feels that his dad has an overpowering sense of helplessness in the face of his son's tragic circumstances. Nevertheless, Kevin and his father are able to talk in detail about what is happening. These conversations have become important sources of support for Kevin. They speak by phone every two or three months and visit in person about every eight months. Kevin has not told his three younger siblings about his illness. He doubts that they know.

Kevin's life-style has changed some since he developed AIDS. He thinks that the changes he has made reflect the changes taking place among gay men in general. Prior to being diagnosed, Kevin had a large number of acquaintances, but it was with his small group of close friends that he spent most of his time. They would visit together at home, go to movies, eat out, or see a play. There were also outings to a bar or elsewhere to meet sex partners. Conversations focused on gay or non-gay political issues, gossip, the arts, bar-based events, or other topics of mutual interest. Kevin's diagnosis has caused him to cease his sexual activity, to engage in more private socializing, to be more attentive to his body and health, and to talk more about depression, fear, isolation, discrimination, and death. Kevin's close friends have become even more important to him. They were told one by one over time what is happening to him. Without exception, the response was supportive and caring. This heartening response, however, paradoxically is painful to Kevin. He is aware of their mutual commitments and the meaning that their friendship gives to his life. His fear of losing them by his death is painful to him.

Equally painful, if not more so, is Kevin's inability to communicate with his mother about what he is experiencing. He is sorry that she is ashamed of him for being gay and having AIDS. But not talking about it burdens both of them even more, in Kevin's opinion. He recalls that she cried when he told her about his homosexuality. She never suspected it. Kevin jokingly remarks: "She must have thought that I was too masculine to be gay. Obviously she never found out that I was trying on her clothes when she was out of the house." Her wish that he had never told her about being gay was a preliminary response consistent with her desire now to avoid more knowledge about her son that is too distressing for her to manage.

Kevin feels as if his life "may be fading away." These feelings are strongest when he is tired, has a headache, or an elevated temperature. He wonders: "Will I get over it; will I be able to do the things that I want before I die; will I ever feel desirable and have an intimate, romantic relationship again; should I make long-term plans; are any but my most immediate plans a waste of precious time; are my frequent, time-consuming trips to the doctors of any value?" Kevin believes that the purple lesions on his skin, although not visible when he is dressed, mark him, that people intuitively know that he has AIDS, and they withdraw. He feels, at times, as if he

73

and his life no longer count. If the data are correct, he will die soon. Why waste time, emotion, and energy on a dead man?

At other times, Kevin has hope. Defiantly he refuses to accept the description of AIDS as an "always fatal" and "terminal" disease. From reading the medical literature about AIDS he is aware that more is being learned all the time. He knows that the life expectancy for people recently diagnosed is better than it is for people diagnosed early in the epidemic. He thinks that the doom-and-gloom terms used in regard to AIDS perpetuate a negativism in patients that becomes a self-fulfilling prophecy. Kevin tries and prefers to think positively. This is why he has not appointed a legal surrogate for himself or made his last will and testament. He has a will to live. He is hopeful that medical science will develop effective treatments or a cure before it is too late for him. Nevertheless, he refuses to be passive about his illness. He presently takes antiviral and immune-boosting drugs that are not approved for nonexperimental use in the United States. He seems to be doing better than some other people he knows with AIDS. Kevin thinks that this may be due to his self-medicating, but he isn't sure. Nevertheless, he feels good about taking an active part in fighting and coping with his disease.

One way in which Kevin copes is through a support group composed of other people with AIDS that he gathered together. They meet regularly to share information, feelings, and concerns. Some of the group's members have become his friends. They met because of AIDS, he explains, but their friendship goes beyond this common trait. AIDS has created some new problems for gay men. But it also has enabled some gay men to let certain qualities or character traits surface. He thinks that many gay men now, with or without AIDS, are becoming more genuine individuals, not merely conformists to expected gay roles and gay behaviors. The aspirations to be a "clone," an indistinguishable part of the crowd, seem to be disappearing. People are realizing that there is precious little time for posturing and playing games. The clock is ticking. Gay men now are doing things together out of compassion and mutual need, rather than out of pity and self-gratification. AIDS has given gay men a reason to grow up, to mature as individuals and as a community.

Another effect of AIDS has been less positive in Kevin's mind. Fear of the disease has become a facade for the expression of latent hatred for and oppression of homosexual people. Fear of AIDS and fear of homosexuality have joined forces to effect an even more powerful, concerted blatant effort to discriminate against and disenfranchise gay and lesbian people. The potentially limiting impact of repressive actions on employment, housing, and insurance options, for example, is frightening to Kevin. His concern is less for himself, since he works as a free-lance writer. He is concerned, nevertheless, for his homosexual brothers and sisters, who fight for their rights, respect, and decent treatment in a hostile environment.

MARY

Mary saw her dream come true only to have it destroyed by the AIDS virus. She is an attractive, softspoken, charming, intelligent young woman. She describes herself as an old-fashioned girl who wanted a husband who would be the man of the house and father of her children. Marriage, family, and home took on an added importance for Mary, since she is an adopted child. Her adoptive parents told her that she was "special." When she was six years old Mary discovered that "special" meant adopted. When the family tree was compiled, her name appeared in the appropriate place. However, the word adopted, within parentheses, was placed behind it. Even though her parents loved her and generously provided for her as a child, she has never felt that she is fully part of them.

Mary initiated a search for her biological parents when she became an adult. Her quest was successful. She discovered that her young mother and father planned to marry. But when the wedding date approached, her father backed out, even though Mary's mother was pregnant with her. Her mother went to a home for unwed mothers, delivered Mary, and put her up for adoption. Although Mary now knows her biological mother and wants to maintain a relationship, her biological mother has refused.

Mary's biological father is a wealthy rancher. When she found him he seemed pleased. As they learned more about each other, her father indicated that she, rather than his other four children, was the one who had turned out like he had hoped. Mary is musically talented and loves the land, animals, and farming. It seemed to Mary that the relationship with her father would endure. But for reasons unknown to Mary, he cut off all contact with her. In Mary's words, "he deserted me a second time." Thus her grief was compounded. Not only did she lose her mother and father early in life, but she lost them later in life as well.

Despite her insecurities with her adoptive parents and the losses of her biological mother and father, Mary was determined to find her place in life, to have a home and family, to have a career, and to be happy. Mary holds a degree in home economics and has additional training in finance and accounting. She worked hard at her job, often ten to twelve hours a day and on weekends. The company rewarded her industry and competency with promotions and salary increases. She climbed the managerial ladder. At twenty-seven she became chief financial officer of a small manufacturing firm. Despite these achievements, her goals of husband and children remained unmet. Then David entered her life.

David worked for the same company as Mary. He had fewer responsibilities and a much lower salary than she. These factors were unimportant to Mary. As they saw more of each other, Mary fell in love. David was divorced. He had custody of his three children. Mary grew to love David's children as much as she loved him. They decided to marry. Because her home would not be large enough for five, they purchased a much larger and more elegant home. Her salary and credit worthiness made this possible.

Mary and David were married on August 10, 1983. It was a lovely ceremony. Her adoptive parents attended. David's children were part of the ceremony. Mary's dream was being realized. The ecstasy of her wedding day lasted for less than twenty-four hours. The next morning Mary was sick and bleeding vaginally. She continued to be ill for six weeks. She did not feel like having intercourse with her new husband during this period. After six weeks David "demanded his rights." Mary tried but the bleeding became heavier. David took her to a hospital, where it was determined that she had miscarried and now had a ruptured uterus. Emergency surgery, during which she received several units of blood, saved her life. Not only was this pregnancy lost, but she was also told that she would not be able to bear children.

Mary recovered from surgery but never regained her

energy. She went back to work, took care of the house, cared for the children and her husband. She complained of fatigue. She sensed that she was not well. Friends thought that she was depressed about losing the baby. Her physicians found nothing to explain her symptoms, even though she was hospitalized numerous times for more thorough testing. Finally, she was referred for psychiatric treatment. Mary knew that she wasn't mentally sick. She knew that something was wrong with her body. Otherwise, she reasoned, she would not be experiencing the flu-like symptoms and recurrent infections.

Mary began to wonder during the six months after her marriage if she could have been infected with the AIDS virus when she received the blood transfusions. She asked her physicians to test her for antibodies to the AIDS virus. They refused. Finally, one of her physicians agreed to do the test during a hospitalization. The physician, with tears in his eyes, told her that the test was positive—she had been infected by the AIDS virus.

During the months that Mary was searching for an explanation for how she felt, her marriage deteriorated. David and Mary argued. He accused her of being a hypochondriac and hysterical. In addition, David decided to quit working so he could spend more time with his children. Mary, however, was expected to provide financial support for the family, do housework, and care for the children. Their financial condition worsened in parallel with Mary's stamina. During one of her hospitalizations, David took Mary's credit cards and purchased expensive gifts for his children. When she returned home, Mary discovered what David had done. She also discovered that David had turned loose her dog that had been with her for five years. Mary was outraged at both behaviors. She searched the neighborhood every night for three weeks until her pet was found. David refused to help. Mary gave up. She packed David's belongings, put them in the garage, barred him from the house, and filed for divorce. Her marriage ended in March 1984, seven months after it began.

Mary's friends slipped away while she was married. Many did not like her husband. Others thought that she was neurotic. Her positive antibody test, unidentified pneumonia, chronic diarrhea, fungal infections, fatigue, night sweats, and fevers invalidate the presumption of neurosis. Mary has ARC. Co-workers and close friends expressed regret and disbelief when it became known that Mary truly is physically sick. She heard comments like, "I can't believe this has happened to someone as sweet as you. You don't deserve this." Offers to help were received. Mary soon discovered, however, that these were empty gestures. The interest and support implicit to them never seemed to find expression. Few people call when she is sick at home. Even fewer people visit her. No one seems willing to talk with her about how she feels about her many losses.

Mary moved back into her original, smaller house. She took bankruptcy because of her husband's financial irresponsibility. Her social life has become quite restricted. She simply does not have enough energy to work and play too. Her work, dog, and home have become increasingly important to her as other things and relationships that she valued slowly have slipped away. The joy of her wedding day became a "steady progression into despair." Over the past thirty months Mary has come to feel that her life is "out of control."

Mary considered suicide before and after she was diagnosed with ARC. Her losses have been staggering—friends, husband, home, hope for children of her own. In short, Mary has lost her dream. In her own words, "take away a person's dream and you take away a person's life." The AIDS virus is chipping away at her dream unrelentingly. Her losses continue to mount. Her boss recently moved her out of her private office into the hall. Mary was asked to begin training another woman, who took over her private office, to do some of Mary's work. This additional blow to her identity, sense of self-worth, and sense of purpose was severe. She considered suicide once again. Mary planned to take her gun and shoot herself. Three thoughts caused her to delay her planned action. First, she questioned if people who commit suicide go to hell. This concern turned out to be of no consequence. Mary says, "I've been there already." Second, Mary worried about what would happen to her beloved dog. Third, she felt that it was important to speak with one of the authors of this book so that her story could be told. Her hope was that more understanding and compassion would be extended to *all* those who were caught in the AIDS crisis. Mary decided against suicide at that time, but she still considers it to be a legitimate alternative to suffering more and more losses.

Mary's adoptive parents, who live about 300 miles away, have been supportive throughout her illness. They call her every other day, and when she is sick they come to be with her. Her dad, a semiretired health care professional, tries to understand all that is happening to her. He does his best to console her. He used to speak of his hatred for gay people. Before Mary was infected, her father thought that AIDS is God's way of wiping out gay people. He speaks this way less often now. Mary thinks that he is growing more sympathetic toward the suffering of all gay people, especially those with AIDS. Mary's mother is equally supportive of her. She has been more expressive than Mary's father of her grief. She told Mary that Mary was the child that she was depending on to take care of her in old age. Now, with Mary's illness, that security is being taken away. The grief of Mary's mother is for herself and for Mary.

ARC has now forced Mary to stop work. She can no longer maintain her home. She has decided to move home, where her parents can help to care for her and her faithful pet. Almost everything Mary valued in life is now gone or going. She fears tomorrow. She foresees no cure. She expresses little hope. She feels lonely and empty. She can't remember the last time she was touched by someone other than her physicians and parents. Her lot, in Mary's view, can only grow worse. She hesitates to reach out to people. She doesn't want to cause them grief by her death. Mary says that she is not afraid of dying. She is, however, afraid that she may die alone because of people's fear of her disease. All she wants, if death is her fate, is to die with as much dignity and grace as possible.

Mary has always believed in God. She believes that she and God are part of each other. Thus, she can have an inner knowledge of God's will and of right or wrong for her. When she miscarried, Mary thought "horrible" things about God. Her anger with God subsided as time passed. When she was diagnosed with ARC her faith in God deepened. Mary believes that God loves humanity. This love is evidenced by the gifts of intelligence and strength that people can call on when they must cope with adversity.

Mary's experience with ARC has helped her to sympathize with all minorities, especially gay men. People with AIDS or ARC, according to Mary, deserve a chance to live. They ought not be preoccupied with guilt about who they are or what they've done. Neither should they continuously search for an answer to the question—

"Why me?" People with AIDS or ARC need to be secure in their relationships, jobs, homes, families, friends, hopes, and dreams. If this were the case, then maybe they would be able to devote their energy to defeat the virus that is destroying their lives. If the virus could be destroyed or neutralized, then the affected people could be revitalized and their dreams could be reconstructed.

PAUL

Paul understands what it means to say that life is full of risks. At age forty-five Paul was diagnosed with AIDS. The blood products that sustain his life as a hemophiliac were the means by which he was infected by the AIDS virus. It is cruelly ironic that the cause of his continued existence, so to speak, may well become the cause of his demise. Paul is deliberate, articulate, goal-oriented, and deeply religious. Like his parents, he is an active participant in the Church of Jesus Christ of Latter-Day Saints. His religious beliefs have shaped his approach to life and, as will be seen in his story, his approach to death.

Paul married within a few years of being graduated from college. He and his wife wanted to have a large family. They have five children between the ages of four and sixteen. Paul has a managerial position in a major financial institution in Texas. In a continuing effort to secure his family's financial future, Paul has worked full time and pursued graduate study at night. All this while keeping time for his wife and children a high priority.

In addition, Paul has been active in the National Hemophilia Foundation. This involvement began in 1977 on the state level. After two years he was elected to serve the foundation on the national level. He has held

several leadership positions in the national organization, making an important contribution to its financial
and structural strength. Paul held an office in the national foundation in 1983, when the discovery was made
that AIDS was linked to a virus transmissible in blood
and blood products. Paul and the foundation considered the relative risks associated with continued use of
blood products that might be contaminated versus discontinuing use of blood products. He felt that it would
not be prudent to substitute the known high risk to
hemophiliacs of no treatment for the unknown risk of
infection with treatment. Further, he thought that by
1983, it was too late to panic. He and others already may
have been infected. So Paul endorsed proposals to
screen blood and ask people in groups at risk for AIDS
voluntarily to refrain from donating blood. Thus, Paul
played a key role in shaping the National Hemophilia
Foundation's policy regarding AIDS and blood products. He has never felt anger or hostility toward any
group at risk for AIDS, e.g., gay men, bisexual men, or
IV drug abusers. This attitude remains even though he
has known eight of the approximately 150 hemophiliacs,
at present, who have contracted AIDS.

In August 1985 Paul's lymph glands swelled. He began to have a persistent cough and his temperature
stayed around 102 degrees for about a month. He suspected that these symptoms were indications that he
would develop AIDS. Two months later his suspicions
were confirmed. Paul was hospitalized, tested, and diagnosed with AIDS. The diagnosis was a "relief" to Paul
because with this knowledge he knew better how to
organize his life. Paul initially felt some frustration and
depression over the realization that some of the things
he hoped to do would not be done. He feels that he has
between six months and two years to live unless effec-

tive therapies are found before long. Given his perceived constraints of time, Paul now wants to focus even more on his family, particularly his children. He wants to be the most help to them that he can and be as good to them as he can. He wants them to remember him as a helping, loving, good father.

Paul understood his risks for AIDS because of his dependency on blood products. He was prepared to run those risks. However, Paul does not want to put his wife's health and life in jeopardy when they have sexual intercourse. He has used condoms since 1983 as a precautionary measure. She shows no indication of infection by the AIDS virus. Neither of them is afraid that Paul's presence in the home and his contact with their children represent any form of contagious threat to the children. They have always been close as a family. Before leaving home for his first hospitalization, Paul called the family together. The children were told of the possibility that he might have AIDS. They talked together again when the diagnosis was confirmed. The children, except for the youngest, seem to understand what is happening to them. One child who does not characteristically like to be held by Paul insisted on sitting in Paul's lap as the implications of Paul's disclosure were discussed.

Everyone's future is uncertain, according to Paul. His is uncertain and probably shorter. In light of this, Paul is preparing for his family's future without him. Making these arrangements is time-consuming. Paul feels an urgency to do them. Nevertheless, he wants to schedule time amid these activities to "sniff the roses in the garden, to enjoy living and loving, rather than thinking solely of my dying." In short, Paul wants to maximize the quality of his time left with his family.

Paul's eldest son has begun to assume greater responsibility around the house. He told Paul that he'd help his mother. Without being asked, and quite out of character, he cleaned the garage. Paul sees his son acting more like an adult now and beginning to assume a fatherly role with his younger brothers and sisters. This pleases Paul. It underscores his confidence that the family will not be destroyed when he is "gone." This confidence makes him less reluctant to "leave."

Paul is acutely aware that the youngest children may not remember much about him. Also, he realizes that he will not be here to counsel the children as they grow up. Finally, he feels that much of his family's history contained in his memory will be lost with his death. Paul considers these states of affairs unacceptable. Thus, he has begun to make audiotapes. He is recording a history of his childhood, work, religious beliefs, and other life experiences. In addition, he is making a tape for each of his children containing the counsel that he thinks each may want, based on his knowledge of his or her personality and needs for character development, as he or she matures. Finally, when his mother and brother visited at Christmas 1985, they jointly produced a four-hour family oral record of their life as a family.

Having AIDS is no "thrill" to Paul. Nevertheless, he feels that if someone is going to have AIDS, he would rather that it be someone who understands the disease and its attendant risks and who is not afraid of the future, i.e., death. This does not mean, however, that Paul is free from grief. He and his wife have talked extensively about what is happening to them. Their conversations identifying expected events in their children's lives have been most painful to him. He grieves missing ceremonies like graduations and marriages, as well as watching the children develop their own identities in careers and associations. He grieves the loss of his plan to move the family to his hometown, where the children could be in touch with their family roots. Paul grieves his inability to unify his family with its extended and historical relatives. Paul's wife also grieves. At times she cries. She realizes that her and the children's future will be drastically altered by AIDS. Her hurt is for Paul, herself, and the children. She is particularly worried about her ability to be solely responsible for the children's care, financially and otherwise.

In some ways having AIDS has been rewarding for Paul. He has received calls, cards, and letters from people that he knows but with whom he has not felt particularly close. The magnitude and sincerity of these expressions of concern and support have been heartwarming. He has discovered that he has more friends and admirers than he thought. His employer and co-workers have been equally attentive. He will be allowed to work as long as he feels he can. Long-distance phone bills are being paid by his company so that he can have as much contact with his family as possible when he is hospitalized. At Christmas 1985 his co-workers sent flowers and cards. In addition, they collected funds to pay for the transportation and lodging for his wife and children to be with him for the holiday. A Christmas basket from his colleagues was delivered to his room. It contained fruit and $600 to help with holiday expenses. Paul is grateful for these expressions of concern. He intends to thank his co-workers when he returns. He intends, as well, to conduct educational sessions about AIDS, how it is spread, and how badly some people with AIDS are treated.

Paul's religious beliefs have helped to shape his response to the advent of AIDS and his personal experience with the disease. He believes that God is aware of what happens in the world and to people. But Paul does not believe that God intervenes to change the course of events. Some of the people in his church have urged him to ask God in prayer to supernaturally alter his probable future. Other people urge him to summon his faith, to let its strength improve his physical condition and save his life. His mother, who sends him a card every day, implies that she thinks God can and will intervene. Paul asks her and the others why God should intervene for him and not others. AIDS, for him, is a part of life. He sees it as a way for him to learn how to cope with illness and death. He is not afraid of "taking that step." Because of this, his mother and others "should be more at peace." Paul does not think that he should be able to escape death because of his belief in God. Rather, his beliefs are there to help him accept the reality of death. He does not feel as if he is being treated unfairly. To the contrary, he is being treated as fairly as everyone else on earth. In his words, "we are all mortal."

Paul wants his death, like his life, to be a learning experience for his children. He believes that the continuity of life and death is being lost in our society as birth and dying have been removed from the home into hospitals. People hear of birth and death, but they seldom observe either and learn from them. Paul and his wife are talking about his dying at home if the children are adequately prepared. Paul envisages his death at home as a way to draw the family together to share an important experience.

Paul's faith and congregation, who have been supportive, are sources of strength and encouragement in troubled times. Nevertheless, he is critical of the reaction of religious communities to AIDS. He thinks that they have been slow to respond compassionately. The clergy have tried to lead their people and minister to patients and families without obtaining adequate data about the disease and the particular problems of people dealing with it, especially the problems of the gay population. Paul decries efforts by certain fundamentalists and other religious groups to make AIDS a means to implement an agenda of social, political, economic, and ecclesiastical discrimination against gay men. He remembers being on a television show about AIDS with Jerry Falwell. Paul speaks with pride about how he rejected Falwell's claim that AIDS came from God as judgment on sinful gay men. In the long run, Paul thinks that the church's apathy and lack of compassion in response to AIDS will be seen as a "dark day" in the history of Christianity.

Paul also has a message for the public. "AIDS is the most recent but not the only example of humanity's need to learn compassion for one's neighbor. In a paradoxical way, AIDS shows us that we are one people. We all have and need blood to live. Sharing blood, this condition for life, has potential to save and to harm. The diseases that may be borne in blood should be a cause for us to come together to combat the destruction and to comfort the one who suffers. We ought not point a finger of blame at any person or group of people. Rather, we should accept all people who suffer, including all people with AIDS. We should recognize all people with AIDS as people in need of compassion and expressions of our brotherhood and sisterhood. In short, no one should be rejected because of a disease, even if the disease is AIDS."

JOHN

John's story breaks from the format used in the three chapters of stories. This change was deliberate. John is a competent scholar and an introspective, analytic person. By reading John's story in his own words, the reader may sense some of the intrapsychic and sociological distress and accommodation that people with AIDS frequently experience.

"One afternoon in the spring of 1985 I donned my nylon shorts and Nike shoes to run seven miles in my usual way. The next afternoon I went to do the same thing and had so much trouble breathing I had to stop after two miles. In two more days I was in a hospital bed. Thus, out of the blue, began the phase of my life I will tell here.

"For present purposes my name is John. I am a thirty-two-year-old white male, very healthy before AIDS and fairly healthy even now. I hold several advanced degrees in my discipline and have been involved in both teaching and research at the college level.

"The history of my disease is uncomplicated enough. My first infection, of a disseminated fungal sort, struck me by surprise about a year ago. After four months of very nasty chemotherapy I experienced a complete clinical cure. All was fine until December 1985, when I was hospitalized with *Pneumocystis carinii* pneumonia. After two weeks of antibiotics I experienced as complete a clinical cure as one is likely to see with this disease. Again I am feeling well. My absolute T_4 lymphocyte (helper cell) count is somewhere in the range of thirty, which constitutes severe immune deficiency.

"Two things make this history somewhat unusual. First is the rapidity and completeness of clinical cure for two severe infections *despite* very suppressed immune function. Second is the fact that at the time I had my first opportunistic infection, it was not included in the criteria used by the Centers for Disease Control (CDC) for AIDS reporting. Thus, although I had a fulminant infection and very low immune function, it was actually some months later that I was officially diagnosed. Needless to say, even without a firm diagnosis I was very worried. Young homosexual men who eat well, run fifty miles a week, lift several thousand pounds of weights per day, get sufficient rest, and so on—such as myself—

just don't come down one day with disseminated disease . . . *unless* they have AIDS. So I lived for several months in great *fear* of the truth before the CDC—mercifully—put a new word on their list of inclusion criteria and I came to *know* the truth. As I tell my story, I won't go into some of what I'm feeling now because a lot of it is very similar to what many people feel when they are faced with a big disappointment and loss. There are already books that tell of such feelings: denial, devaluation, and so on. In these ways I feel I must have been created from a rib of Elisabeth Kübler-Ross. I want you to know about some of my special experiences.

"The biggest thing going on with me right now is a sort of compulsive anxiety. I am experiencing such angst I feel I should be a character in a German expressionist play. A big source of this unease is the sheer fact that I am now operating with a deadline (no pun intended). Many people who are faced with deadlines endure a lot of anxiety in meeting them. However, most such people are at least roughly aware of *when* the deadline will be reached. My deadline, on the other hand, is a surprise deadline. I have no way of anticipating its arrival, or of using such information to assist me in prioritizing my life. So I often find myself trying to do everything that I ever want to accomplish at once. Nobody can work that way.

"I can't tell what's important any more. Every goal, every ideal, every value I ever held is now jumbled with every other in a big heap. On optimistic days everything seems important. On pessimistic days nothing seems important. On most days I am somewhere in between, permuting every commitment of my life with nothing solid to hang on to.

"I've always swung between idealistic and cynical extremes; my mental life has been a tension between the role models of Mohandas K. Gandhi and H.L.

Mencken. At some time I have found myself balanced at almost every intermediate point. AIDS has just made it harder for me to stay in one place for any length of time.

"Since my pneumonia I've been more compulsive than ever, and on many more levels. For example, with respect to my relationship to my environment, I have experienced the following: (1) I now notice *everything*. Good, bad, happy, sad: I notice it all. Flowers, sunsets, crippled old people, potholes in the streets. Everything is elevated to the level of conscious awareness. Much of it would have passed unnoticed a short while ago. This level I call my Noticer. (2) I now place a moral/aesthetic/ humorous/cynical evaluation on everything I notice. Thus, data proceeds from the Noticer to the Evaluator. Many of these evaluations are very elaborate, requiring much theoretical support. (3) Once the Evaluator has done its job, the Printer is eager to kick in. I want to *tell* someone all about it, or *write* a letter to someone. Not just anyone will do, of course. The recipient of my output must be someone I consider capable of fully appreciating the morality or the aesthetics or humor, etc. At times it is hard to find such a listener, especially one who has time to listen. So the Printer is frustrated frequently. I am, happily, beginning now to get a grip on these three levels—especially the Printer and the Evaluator. Don't get me wrong. I don't think these are bad developments—indeed the contrary. But one can have too much of any good thing, and so I am pleased to be beginning to assign a proper place to the three levels of verbal compulsiveness.

"Compulsiveness can hit at other levels as well. At the very same time I am becoming more verbal and ex-pressive than I've ever been, I am also siphoning a lot of energy into being nice to people. So many people have been so nice to me since my disease began that I now want to be nice to everybody. It isn't a feeling of obligation out of gratitude so much as a remembrance of how *good* others' kindness made me feel. And being nice takes many forms. I can help a friend move his whole household of furniture or I can smile and say 'Good morning' to the lady running the elevator. Being nice comes in all degrees. At any degree, though, being nice requires some investment—however small or large—of my time, effort, or whatever. Even common courtesy requires a small sacrifice. I must take a little time away from my own thoughts and projects in order to do something as simple as holding a door open for someone. Thus, being compulsive about being nice can often be at odds with being compulsive about my own work. Shall I linger to chat with this acquaintance out of friendship, or shall I hustle back to the typewriter to finish my AIDS vignette?

"One reason for my compulsiveness in being nice to people now is precisely my agnosticism concerning any divine arbiter who will some day set all wrongs right. I have lived most of my life in a way that was *not* very nice for other people. Since I do not think this fault will be corrected on any cosmic scale, I am now compelled to try to set it right myself—and in a hurry.

"I wonder if much of my compulsiveness lately is out of insecurity. Perhaps I am afraid that my passing will not be adequately grieved. That people won't fully appreciate what they're losing when they lose me. I have wished that there could be a little adhesive strip somewhere in this book with my name written under it. Then, after I'm gone and anonymity requirements are moot, everyone could pull off the strip and know that *I* wrote this.

"The contradictions of my life have become glaring. One day last week I wrote to the Hemlock Society for help in planning my death and paid a travel agent for tickets to Mexico where I must go to purchase an experimental drug that may save my life. Death and life, black and white. I am caught up in a vortex somewhere in between.

"Recently there have been flashes of insight in which my whole life and mind seem transparent to me. I am like a glass layer cake. The layers at the top are just specialized and elaborately decorated versions of those at the bottom. Perhaps we are not as complex as we think—or perhaps we are more so.

"The mailbox brought good news and bad today. The good news is that my father mailed me a check for $200. The bad news is that my latest hospital bill arrived— $8,000. Easy come, easy go. Things like money and credit don't bother me as much any more as they used to. I once became extremely guilty and ashamed when I would receive a late notice from the bank or other creditor. No human being was even aware that I had been sent the notice, since it is all computerized, but still I reacted as if I had stolen something. Now, though, things are different. I pay when I am well enough to work, and I let the bills slide when I am not. I don't let it bother me like it used to. One day it occurred to me that the only reason to be overcautious about your finances is that someday in the future you may again need credit. But when you have no *future* in which to need credit, you have less reason to be financially meticulous.

"In fact, this feeling of liberation from much that conventionally constrains people in society is one of the truly positive aspects of my experience with AIDS. In many ways I am now more relaxed than I've ever been before simply because when you're about to lose everything, the loss of any particular thing is not cause for much concern.

"I've been thinking a lot about forgiveness of late. I guess there is a part of me that is still feeling guilty about my homosexuality. That part of me needs to be

93

forgiven—most of all by *me*. I have tormented myself with guilt about sex since I was a little boy. It has gotten in the way of having any pleasure in most of the sexual encounters I have had in my life. I always liked thinking and, later, talking about sex better than having it because I didn't feel as much guilt with the former. I always liked masturbation better than contact with another person because masturbation, though shameful, was not *as* shameful. Another man, another masturbation fantasy. The sooner you flush him down the toilet, the sooner you can stop feeling inadequate and start your guilt trip. This is one of the ironies of *my* having AIDS: I never got enough pleasure from sex in any form to deserve to pay this price. Of course, I *know* that neither AIDS nor any other disease is the sort of thing that can be deserved by anyone. But I cannot help what I *feel*, despite what I know.

"I was never as promiscuous as many gay men are, but I did have my little coming-out party. Unfortunately, the AIDS virus was coming out about the same time I was. Now I find it difficult to feel terribly ashamed of my own one-time promiscuity or about gay promiscuity in general. Our society makes us hide this important part of ourselves and denies us open access to more conventional ego strokes. So we take to the sheets. We are people who have been told by their culture to do certain things (like become a success) without being given what we need to accomplish them (like self-respect). It is hard to build a mansion when you must live in a closet.

"Just after I had my first opportunistic infection I met a wonderful man, Gene. Gene is very intelligent and sensitive and represents a good complement to my own personality. We can help each other grow as people because we are alike and different. I love Gene and he loves me very much. In general I am very much happier now that I know him than I have ever been before. But we can't have certain forms of physical contact because of my problem. This generates a lot of worry and grief for both of us. There are so many ironies associated with AIDS, and my difficulties with Gene help to point up one of them. Before we began taking AIDS seriously, gay men were very promiscuous, by and large. Then came AIDS and we all got scared and cut down on our sexual activity. And lo, we found that the men we had always seen as mere sexual-gratification devices are real *people*. We discovered that you can get your ego stroked by another man without having your penis stroked. You can make friends and party together and have a very good time without going to bed. You can even, if you are very lucky, find a wonderful person with whom you want to settle down for a very long time. Then you find out *you* have AIDS. The disease that helped us to live more fully now threatens to take *your* life.

"Many people find many of my current attitudes and behaviors peculiar, given the circumstance of my disease and what it portends. For example, just because I got sick I did not stop having my head turned by a pretty face. Nor did I stop commenting to my friends about how hot I considered a given passerby to be. I did not stop being a sexual being with deep sexual needs just because I got a (predominantly) venereal disease. I am *very* conscientious about refraining from any kind of activity that might expose anyone else to what I've got; but I like to *talk* about doing fun things with the hot guys I see even if I can't *do* them any more. Sometimes, though, I don't feel worthy even to think about having a sexual interlude with anybody. I often feel dirty. I often perceive myself as being so much thinner, less toned, and older-looking than I was before that I cannot even bring myself to fantasize about somebody attractive wanting to have sex with me.

"Some people, especially some of my closest friends,

are horrified by my often 'sick' and sardonic humor vis-à-vis my condition. They must think I'm being very cavalier, but really I'm not. It's just another way of coping. And anyway, would they rather laugh with me or cry with me?

"Physically, I appear very well; yet I am *very* sick. My immune function is perhaps among the lower 10 percent of the clinic population who constitute my fellow AIDS sojourners. But I look fit and robust and in the pink of health. I am very happy about this contradiction, because if I *looked* as bad as my immunity *is*, I'd be breaking mirrors all over town. Nevertheless, even healthy looks have their drawbacks. I feel at times like nobody takes my disease seriously because they look at me and I look fine. And I'm not talking just about my friends. The doctors in the clinic also often give me this impression. As if to be really sick you have to be gasping for breath or dwindling to eighty pounds.

"I've never told my parents that I'm gay; even now, they think I have cancer, not AIDS. They may suspect, but we've never talked about it. They both live in smaller communities where gay men are seldom seen or thought of: kids at play, suburban lawns. In the past I have enjoyed brief trips to these communities because I could act out a guilt fantasy of being straight. I now have the additional pleasure of enacting a fantasy of being healthy.

"Straight people, whether in large communities or small, don't think about homosexual people very much. So they don't think much about AIDS. This is part of why not enough is being done. But we grow up and we grow old. We feel joy and we feel pain. We work hard and we try at every turn to be the very best people we can. Just like everybody else. We have so much in common with other people it is incredible that we allow ourselves to be divided over whom we like to sleep with.

"My greatest fears at present are losing Gene, losing my mind, getting Kaposi's sarcoma, becoming debilitated and dependent, having my parents become disappointed in me. These fears and others are interspersed with great and small joys, as well as considerable hope.

"Things I feel luckiest about: I have not been abandoned by my friends, by my family, by Gene. I look and feel pretty well most of the time. My employer has been very understanding and helpful financially. Sven, my therapist, has been very generous with his time. My doctors in the clinic are among the best in the world for people in my condition. I am perhaps happiest about all the growing up which this disease has made me do in a short time. I have learned organization and efficiency. I have learned that a creative project doesn't have to be perfect before it is good enough to let others see it. I have learned to pay attention to much more of what is going on around me, especially things that involve people and their feelings.

"Something I am not particularly worried about: being dead. Ways of dying—and ways of living—*are* things that can be feared. But the state of being dead is not a problem for me.

"I have helped to provide care to some guys who experienced terrifying ways of dying with AIDS. I am resolved to avoid such an experience for myself and so have considered ways of self-destruction. To continue to live when life has become a hopeless tragedy is both irrational and wrong. The trick is knowing when you have reached this bridge. There are no signposts along the way. You must hope that your body will let you know while you yet have time and strength to take matters into your own hands.

"I apologize to the reader for the somewhat disjointed style of this piece. But my life is now disjointed, and the piece *is* about me. As far as I am concerned, I am going to survive this disease, thanks partly to my very strong and resilient body, partly to my having enough sense to know how to take care of myself, and partly to other people: my friends, my doctors, the scientists who are working for a cure. So the present piece is more a report of work in progress than an auto-obituary.

"After death we live on, if at all, as memories. We hope that we will be well remembered by the people whom we touched in life. They will downplay the bad and emphasize the good. It is possible, too, that we shall all live on eternally as memories in the mind of God. There, God will perform a great miracle and cause himself to forget all our wickedness. For God is a forgiving God, and perfect forgiveness must be forgetful. Thus cleansed, we shall be well remembered indeed."

Families and Lovers

4

THELMA AND RALPH

Ralph was twenty-five years old when he experienced a second conversion. Brought up by devout parents in the Church of God in Christ, he had confessed his faith and was baptized at the age of sixteen. Now, as he reflected on his new experience, he dedicated his life anew and sought training as a pastor. His three years in one of the church's colleges excited him and confirmed his sense of call to the ministry. When he finished training he presented himself to be called to a congregation. He was baffled to find that his call was not accepted by those from whom he sought endorsement. He struggled with this situation for months and reluctantly resigned himself to the judgment that his call lay in other directions.

Now married, and with a growing family, he became an active member of a Church of God in Christ congregation in a mid-sized city in central Oklahoma. He was elected deacon and quickly assumed leadership positions in the congregation, ultimately being named superintendent of the Sunday school. Within five years it was one of the largest school programs within the church's jurisdiction. He and his wife, Thelma, saw that their four children were brought up in the church. Ralph loved each of them but reserved his most secret hopes for his only son. In his heart he gave Ralph Jr. to God, praying that his son might have opportunities denied to himself. Following employment opportunities in another city, Ralph Sr. found new opportunities in a newly established congregation in his new location. The whole family quickly became involved in its life, the three girls singing in the junior choir and Ralph Jr. accepting leadership in the youth fellowship. Their father began the task of organizing the church school, and under his leadership it grew quickly beyond the physical capacities of the buildings. The congregation enthusiastically expanded the church plant to house the adult classes.

Ralph Sr. began to experience growing problems with the leadership of the congregation. A family decision was made to leave the church and join an independent congregation nearby. Throughout these years he continued to treasure the hope that his son would experience the same call that he had felt as a young man. Ralph Jr. gave no indication that he felt a call to the ministry, although he continued to play an active part in the life of the church. He seemed to enjoy the usual patterns of dating young women, but the relationships never matured. He had chosen architecture as a career and proved to be an effective administrator, with gifts in interior design. He benefited from a number of promotions in the firm that had hired him, achieving staff status in an unexpectedly short time. Ralph Sr. was proud of his son, and his anxiety that his success might draw him away from the church proved unfounded. Ralph Sr. and Thelma found much satisfaction in the close relationships that characterized their family life, which now included the daughters' husbands and growing grandchildren. That degree of closeness, although they may not have been consciously aware of its meanings, compensated them for earlier disappointments.

At the age of fifty-three Ralph suffered the first of two heart attacks. He hovered between life and death for three weeks. His first conscious thought in the coronary ICU (intensive care unit) was a prayer that God would spare him to give him time to meet his obligations as a husband and a father. He was confident that he would be "given a miracle." Had not God already made a miraculous intervention in their lives when his youngest daughter survived when born with a congenital heart abnormality that was usually considered fatal? He returned to health, only to suffer a second attack three years later. It was not as serious as the first, and Ralph Sr. never faltered in his conviction that God was watching over him. He knew in his heart that God had still more work for him to do. It was while he was recovering from the second attack that the company for which he had worked all his life was acquired by a larger organization, and the new owner began to lay off the older workers. He was fortunate. His employment continued through 1983, when he was offered an attractive separation bonus for early retirement. He agreed to retire, but his life was suddenly clouded by another anxiety. For some years he had been aware that Ralph Jr. had restricted his friends to young men his own age. He had his suspicions but hid from Thelma his concern that their son was homosexual. She had enough worries of her own because of his own ill health and the everyday care of a growing family.

In January 1983 Ralph Jr., then aged thirty-three years, informed his parents that he is gay and introduced them to Rob, with whom he was then living. Ralph Sr. and Thelma struggled to accept his life-style, turning to their religious upbringing for guidance. The guidance was mixed. They both came from families with strong Puritan influences and had sought to communicate those values to their children. They could not approve of the nature of their son's relationship with Rob, but they did not swerve from their acceptance of them as people. They took literally the injunction that they should not judge, lest they be judged themselves. Ralph was still their son, and as parents, they remembered the story of the prodigal, whose father did not ask what he had done in the far country, but ran and threw his arms around him and welcomed his return as a full member of the family. Ralph Sr. turned more and more frequently to family relationships for his source of reassurance. He found relief in the manner in which his daughters and their husbands continued to accept Ralph Jr. and Rob. He found that Ralph's sisters had known about Ralph's sexual identity and had accepted his judgment that it would only hurt their parents if that was disclosed to them. This knowledge now confronted Ralph Sr. with a new concern. How would the members of their congregation respond if they learned the family's secret? With Ralph living across town, he had been worshiping in another congregation. Now that his parents knew of his life-style, he frequently accompanied them to church. They decided to say nothing to their pastor or their fellow members.

In June 1983 Ralph Jr. became ill with a series of infections that his parents learned two months later had been diagnosed as the onset of AIDS. At the same time Rob began to develop similar symptoms, and in November 1983 both were hospitalized. By this time Ralph's retirement had become effective, and he spent his days with Ralph Jr. at the hospital, leaving only when Thelma or one of the daughters was able to relieve him. After a series of crises, Ralph's condition began to stabilize and he was discharged. Rob remained in hospital, and Ralph Sr. displayed the same care for Rob that he had shown for his son. He noted that Rob's parents visited him each day and learned that they had taken an apartment in town for that purpose. Ralph Jr. returned to his parents' home temporarily, so that Thelma could provide the constant care he then needed.

It was impossible for Ralph Jr. to keep the nature of his illness from his administrator at work, as members of the staff visited him in hospital. It was not long before his diagnosis was common knowledge. At first his employment did not appear threatened. His staff position in the firm was secure, and in May 1984 he was given the responsibility of opening and managing a new company office. He successfully completed his assignment and expected that his work would be recognized with an appropriate promotion and salary increase. He was shattered when he learned that the entire team of seven whom he had supervised on a recently completed project received commendations and raises, but that his own salary was frozen. His parents shared his bitterness and began to recognize that community attitudes were hardened and unforgiving. It did not seem to matter that Ralph's work for the firm was above reproach. They watched helplessly as time and again Ralph Jr. suffered hurt and humiliation at the hands of his fellow staff members. It seemed as if the firm itself assumed that his death was inevitable and was prepared to "wait him out." Ralph stunned his parents with the announcement that the firm had "marked him off as dead already."

Ralph Sr. reflected on his own situation. Brought up in the Puritan tradition of three generations in a family that rejected homosexuals as unacceptable to God, he nevertheless did not waver in his support of his son. He and Thelma continued to support both Ralph and Rob, providing medical care under the supervision of the men's physician and accompanying them on visits to the hospital's outpatient clinics. While still feeling defensive and protective, Thelma and Ralph were at peace with themselves, although that peace was constantly threatened by their growing awareness of the course of AIDS in its victims' lives. Their job, they believed firmly, was to help Ralph and Rob to keep their positive attitude as a means of fending off the inevitable periods of depression that accompanied each new crisis.

Ralph and Thelma had decided long ago that they could not share their family's pain with their pastor. They did not believe that he would understand their decisions. They did not expect him to do so, but in any case they could not risk the matter becoming generally known throughout the congregation. Ralph Jr. had been hurt enough! Their son resolved the issue by discontinuing to worship with them and joining an Episcopal church. He told them that he had found a real sense of peace in the daily communion service that he attended on his way to work. He had begun to drop into the church building in the late afternoon when the quietness of the empty building intensified his feeling of communion with God. For his parents, Ralph's decision was both a source of peace and a reminder that they were without the religious support of their own church community, a decision that they have not felt able to change.

Ralph's life since contracting AIDS has been marked by persistent episodes of *P. carinii* infections, causing intermittent hospitalizations, and regular outpatient clinic visits for chemotheraphy treatments. On one occasion Ralph and Rob were accompanied by their parents for a planned meeting with the medical team that was treating them. Their physician informed them that they were becoming a medical puzzle, since they had survived a series of infections that they had not been expected to overcome. Ralph Sr.'s response to this statement startled the physician, whom he informed that God had already given the family miracle after miracle, and he expected God to act again to restore his son and Rob to health. Bravely as he made the statement, he also knew that most of his son's acquaintances had already died of AIDS. Yet how else could their apparent recovery from one infection after another be understood? Ralph Jr. attempted to warn his father against unrealistic expectations, while appreciating his need for assurance and wishing to shelter him as much as possible. Ralph Sr. found his greatest reassurance in a later conversation with his son, when Ralph informed him that he found an inner peace through his conversion to the Episcopal Church. In his words, "I prayed about it, Daddy, and I believe it was the only thing I could do, where I could get someone to accept me. I now have a place where I belong." As Ralph Sr. contemplated that conversation, he looked and said quietly: "I gave him back to God years ago, and God looks after his own."

MARY AND FRANK

Keith's parents remember their son's graduation from college with the typical quiet reserve of an East Texas farming family. Keith had grown up on the edge of the Big Thicket, learning as a boy to hunt, to know and live with nature, and to act responsibly as a caretaker of its resources. His parents' reserve at graduation could not mask their pride in Keith's achievements. Their home bore testimony to Keith's active involvement in a wide variety of extracurricular activities. They had been strict with both of their children, but Keith was the elder child and the only son. Looking back now they could not imagine making any substantive changes in the way they had related to their children. Now those memories and Keith's accomplishments are their only consolation.

Keith had attended Southern Methodist University, majoring in math and physics. Graduating in 1968 with honors, he obtained employment with one of the multi-national contractors of the National Aeronautics and Space Administration, where he began to specialize in computer analysis. His rapid rise in the company's computer department led to a well-paying position with excellent job security. It was not the matter of their son's "success" that led to his parents' deep sense of satisfaction—although they shared his pride of achievement. Their deepest concern had always been issues of values arising out of deeply held religious convictions. It was their awareness that Keith shared these values that caused them to be thankful. They were themselves respected members of their community, including the congregation in which they are active participants. They frequently made the long drive to Houston to visit Keith and invariably did so on his birthday. They always felt close to him, and he returned their love.

They returned to East Texas with considerable anxiety after celebrating Keith's fortieth birthday. They had found him ill, and he had brushed the matter off with the comment that he was suffering from a heavy cold. Five weeks later he called to inform them that he felt much worse and was unable to drive to work, although he was able to complete his responsibilities once he reached his office. They came to Houston, remaining to care for him, driving him to and from work, and preparing his meals. Two weeks after their arrival Keith informed them that he was gay and had been diagnosed as having AIDS.

They were distressed by his statement but decided immediately that their relationship with Keith was in no way changed. During the last three months of his illness they accompanied him to the hospital for treatments and nursed him at home until his final admission before his death. Apart from their deep anguish as he lost weight and the Kaposi's lesions spread, their strongest feeling was the degree of isolation they experienced. After only a brief discussion they were in full agreement that the nature of Keith's illness could not be disclosed to family members, friends, or their pastor. They believed that they knew their community well enough to be convinced that these people would neither understand nor be tolerant toward them.

Perhaps the deepest shock they experienced occurred during a brief visit to their East Texas community, when, passing through a nearby community, they read a church sign bearing the words: *God "AIDS" the Gays.* Many of their neighbors would have approved of the sign. To Mary and Frank it was an affront, both in the light of their own faith in a loving God and their fear for Keith's life. They wanted to protect Keith from their neighbors and congregation, but their action was also self-protective. One result of their decision, however, was that it left them without access to support from the very community—neighbors and congregation—to which they ordinarily would have turned. Gradually, as they made their own peace with their situation, they informed a few trusted family members and friends, all of whom lived outside their own community. When it was necessary to speak about Keith's illness, it was in terms that he had cancer and was not responding to therapy.

This decision created a deep feeling of unease for Mary and Frank. They had never resorted to lying to mask their handling of difficult situations. Now they found themselves withholding the truth from their pastor and closest friends, and it weighed on their minds.

They found comfort from only two avenues. Keith's social worker reassured them that it was not inaccurate to refer to his illness as a cancer, and arrangements were made to denote that as the cause of death. Had the death certificate read otherwise, they dreaded the news reaching their community through the agency of the funeral home. They sought further protection by arranging interment in a small, little-used cemetery some distance from their hometown.

Reflecting on these events some months after Keith's death, in October 1985, Frank recalled a second source of consolation. During the time they spent with Keith while he was in hospital, they found a community of support in the parents of other AIDS patients. One family in particular had sought treatment in a community far from their own in Michigan. With few exceptions these families had decided to withhold information from pastors and congregations for reasons similar to those of Frank and Mary. They did not wish to expose themselves and their families to the stigma that they were painfully aware most people applied to the illness and its victims. Each family chose to accept the isolation as the least painful of their options.

Frank and Mary were adamant about one issue: they never felt alienated from their son. "If we had to do it over again," Frank stated, "we would do exactly the same." As for Keith's life-style, which was very different from their own, they remain puzzled. They do not understand why Keith was gay. He had often brought girls home to meet them, both while in college and later. They wished that they had been able to discuss it with him. But by the time he decided to disclose to them his sexuality, his mind was already affected by the virus, and they never learned the whole story. They loved Keith deeply. And they miss him.

FRANCES AND TOM

Frances remembers how the phone call interrupted their sleep, and their lives. For the past few days they had been reviewing plans that Tom was formulating to accept a new contract that would set his small company on its feet. It would require some sacrifices for a while, and he wanted to be sure that Frances was fully versed in its details and its implications for their lives. They were both in their second marriage, moving to Texas when the opportunity to start the new company arose. Tom's college-age daughter, Ruth, was living with them, and the relationship pleased Frances. Her only son, Bryan, lived in New Jersey and flew home often to visit them. He and his stepsister were close friends. This also was a source of satisfaction. Bryan was not her only child. His younger brother had been killed in an airplane crash at the age of twenty-three. The constant awareness of that tragedy tempered her joy and sometimes threatened her peace of mind. At such times she turned to her parish priest and the offices of the church for strength. Her own inner strength and vitality had carried her through many crises, but she knew that these were often not enough on their own.

The hospital caller informed her that Bryan had been rushed to hospital with pneumonia and was asking for her. She flew to New Jersey on the first morning flight. For the next two months Frances lived in Bryan's hospital room. The first major complication followed an adverse reaction to medication, extending what should have been a brief hospitalization to eight weeks. During that period Bryan's lover, Timothy, maintained his relationship with Bryan through hospital visits, care of Bryan's dog, bringing mail, and so forth. Frances welcomed Tim, making it clear that she accepted his presence and his ministration to Bryan. It became apparent to Frances, however, that Tim resented her involvement with Bryan, especially her constant presence in the hospital room. Only when they were away from Bryan did Tim request Frances directly to leave. This she refused to do, stating that she would only consider returning home if Bryan made the request. Tim grew increasingly sharp with her, leading to a final scene in which he insisted that he wanted an exclusive relationship with Bryan. Tim felt that he should be regarded as Bryan's next of kin. Frances was prepared to accept this arrangement only if Bryan asked her to leave. She was happy to include Tim in all discussions and arrangements, but until Bryan decided otherwise, she was legally Bryan's next of kin. Tim thereupon removed his belongings from Bryan's apartment and made no further attempt to contact Bryan. Toward the end of the hospital stay, Frances called her husband to ask whether he would accept Bryan into their home. Without hesitation, Tom responded: "This is Bryan's home. Bring him home." Frances learned later that, on hearing the nature of his stepson's illness, Tom had gone to a medical library and read all the material he could find on AIDS. By the time Frances and Bryan returned from New Jersey, Tom knew much of what was known on the subject. He knew also that knowledge was changing almost daily. Shortly after arriving in Texas, Bryan was hospitalized after a severe reaction to a new antibiotic, spending the next ten weeks in hospital. Other periods as an inpatient followed, interspersed with almost daily trips to outpatient clinics for chemotherapy. Among the complications that seemed now to be never-ending, Bryan developed "chemical diabetes" owing to a further drug reaction.

Frances had known that Bryan is gay since his nineteenth birthday. She had cried the whole day that she was told. Then she decided that this was a discovery Bryan had made, and that she would have to live with it. Once that decision had been made, she put the issue behind her and expected others to accept Bryan as her son. With the death of her younger son her relationship with Bryan became even more important. She was saddened after her return from New Jersey to find that Ruth refused to enter the house. She attributed her decision to the danger of contracting AIDS, despite growing medical evidence that she was not at risk and her awareness that her father was participating equally in caring for Bryan, for example, assisting him to bathe and including him in the hugs by which family members expressed their affection. Frances often wondered if Ruth's attitude was influenced by the fact that she was engaged to a "red-neck." Frances worked hard at maintaining her own relationship with Ruth, being particularly careful to share in the planning and excitement of her forthcoming marriage.

One of the most poignant moments during the long period of Bryan's illness occurred when Bryan and Tom were watching TV one evening. Bryan asked his stepfather if he would be willing to adopt him. Tom replied that adoption was something that usually happened when children were young and was hardly necessary for Bryan, now aged twenty. Bryan appeared discouraged. When the issue was pressed, Tom realized belatedly how important it was to him. He responded cheerfully that he was privileged Bryan should seek this step. He would be pleased to inquire about what steps needed to be taken. Once that issue had been resolved, Bryan did not raise the matter again. Frances and Tom began to recognize that it was not the issue of taking steps for formal adoption that concerned Bryan, but the question of whether Tom and Frances were prepared to entertain the possibility. With Tom's positive response to his request, Bryan had received the answer he sought. He seemed to settle down, with little evidence of the agitation that had begun to characterize his prolonged stay. He was a member of the family, and therein found his peace.

There was no question of Bryan returning to New Jersey. He remained on his company's payroll, but on extended leave. He qualified for the appropriate medical assistance available to a totally disabled person by maintaining his New Jersey apartment, thereby meeting residency requirements. Two needs were thus met. First, Bryan could still talk of having his own residence and, to that extent, continue to think of himself as an independent person. His family could see that this was important to him. Second, during the period before Bryan's loss of abilities owing to the viral attack on his central nervous system, one of his constant themes had been the frequency with which families of people with AIDS had rejected patients, including refusing to provide shelter. With the deterioration in his mental awareness, Bryan no longer appeared to be alarmed by the possibility, but his earlier apprehension was not forgotten by either Tom or Frances.

When asked if she had discussed with Bryan the fatal consequences of contracting AIDS, Frances responded that not only had she *not* raised the subject of dying and death, but spoke always of Bryan's return to health. Right or wrong, she and Tom had decided that this was the only way to maintain any semblance of hope in Bryan, particularly during periods when the adverse drug reactions were so overwhelming. More recently, his failing mental status rendered the matter moot. The only point at which the question was even remotely raised was through a discussion that led Bryan to give Frances power of attorney over his affairs. Even then the deeper issues were skirted. "Now, what difference can it make?" Frances asked.

Bryan spends his days lying on the sofa in the den, watching the afternoon soaps, the family dog nestled beside him, and with Frances going about her housework, involving him as much as possible in the family's daily activities. She still talks about his recovery but knows the possibilities are slight. Her strength lies in her family relationships and her faith. Her parish priest is important to her because Bryan is important to him. He is warm and sensitive, supporting Bryan and her by visits to their home in priestly ministry, which has included the sacramental offices of the Eucharist and Anointing of the Sick. With that foundation, Frances says quietly, she can face anything.

CHARLES

Charles was the lover of Richard, whose story was told in the previous chapter. As noted there, Charles and Richard became lovers in 1981. The condominium that they purchased together was to be an interim home while careers were pursued. After seven or ten years they thought that they would be able to afford the sort of house that both of them wanted as a permanent home. Even so, they began to put their "touch" on the condominium. Richard, being the one with aesthetic sensitivities in the family, assumed primary responsibility for the selection of colors, furniture, fabrics, and wall pieces. Because he also was a handyman, Richard connected their sound system, television, and videocassette recorder. Speakers were strategically placed throughout the house. Every room was transformed into a sound chamber. Further, Richard began to remodel the kitchen and bathrooms. Charles worked long hours managing a retail store. He was relieved from sharing in these duties. Charles' absence was probably an advantage, since he was not too good with his hands, either as a craftsman or as a cook.

Richard did almost all the cooking and much of the housework. He enjoyed doing it all. He was happy being with Charles. The division of labor was unimportant. He was pleased to see Charles doing so well in his career. When time allowed, Charles and Richard would go to a movie, a concert, or the theater. As their careers consumed more time they pursued these leisurely activities more infrequently. They also had less time and energy to make love. Sex had become a minor part of their relationship six months before Richard began to have symptoms of AIDS.

Charles never told his father and stepmother that he is gay. His parents knew that he had a roommate; no other explanations were requested or given. Richard wanted Charles to be honest with his parents about their relationship. Charles, however, did not consider it necessary. They lived 1,500 miles away. When they visited twice a year sleeping arrangements were altered anyway. Each of Charles' three brothers and two sisters knew that Charles is gay and Richard was his lover. They affirmed Charles and approved of Richard. They agreed with Charles that their devoutly Roman Catholic parents should not be told until there was a need for them to know.

Charles told his brothers and sisters about Richard's diagnosis of AIDS. They were supportive. Phone calls, cards, and letters regularly were received. Richard was treated as one of the family. Charles' parents were told that Richard had cancer. They, too, were quick to respond affirmatively, always asking about him and offering to help as they could. However, Charles and

Richard asked for nothing material, only their emotional support and prayers.

Charles was twenty-four when Richard was diagnosed. He, like Richard, was shocked by the news. He wondered if Richard had been infected by him. Charles came out when he was nineteen. He soon settled into a relationship with a man about the same age. They were faithful to each other during their relationship, which lasted for eighteen months. Charles dated some after the breakup. By the time he met Richard he had had a total of six sex partners in three years. Nevertheless, he was concerned about what he possibly had done to Richard and he worried if he, too, would become ill.

These concerns were secondary to Charles' commitment to Richard. Although he was the younger of the two, Charles felt that he had to be strong for Richard. He would constantly tell Richard that "they" would "beat this." He promised never to leave him; they had heard that many lovers of men with AIDS had done so. Charles' anger and fear were carefully masked in Richard's presence with optimism, resolve, and strength. Charles' tears were kept secret from Richard. Their reliance on each other grew as Richard's disease progressed. Their life together before AIDS was somewhat private. They did not wish to "throw open the windows and doors to their lives when Richard got AIDS. It was happening to them, not everyone they knew." So only a few friends were told. Fewer still could endure the strain and be faithful to them until the end. Charles began to love Richard more than ever before, partly because he felt that Richard would die and partly because he felt that he had to make up for the love that other people were withdrawing.

The stresses to Richard and Charles of AIDS were constant and cumulative. Early optimism faded as more and more complications developed. Their anger and frustration with the disease took its toll on each of them and their relationship. Near the end Richard's moods changed frequently and radically. Charles never knew what to expect when he arrived home from work. Richard could be happy and playful, or he could be sad and withdrawn, he could be sick, or he could be dead. Rather than face what was becoming more and more stressful, Charles stayed at the store later and later. Subconsciously, Charles believes in retrospect, he was physically and emotionally distancing himself from Richard and the death that looked more and more probable.

The most painful experience for Charles occurred the summer before Richard died. Richard's eyesight was failing. Neurological problems impaired his memory and coordination. The independence that he valued so highly was being taken from him by these complications. Charles would find food on the stove that Richard overlooked or forgot to put away. Splashes of salad dressing, for example, on the kitchen wall were evidence of Richard's frustration and anger about not being able to care for himself. Richard complained that by the time he finished reading instructions on a food package he had forgotten them.

Richard awoke one Sunday morning in a particularly good mood. Charles worked on Sundays from 11 A.M. to 3 P.M. Richard volunteered to let Charles sleep later while he prepared breakfast. Charles heard Richard cursing loudly and throwing cooking utensils around the kitchen. He could not coordinate his movements to prepare an omelet. Charles went to the kitchen, told Richard to go sit down, that he would prepare breakfast. Richard belligerently refused. Charles snapped, grabbed weak, defenseless Richard, pushed him against the wall, and screamed, "You can destroy your life and our relationship, but you're not going to destroy our home." At that moment Charles realized that Richard in fact would die. Richard could not resist him physically and he could not resist his disease either. The anger that Charles had kept inside exploded at last. His anger was multifaceted—AIDS, Richard, effect on their relationship, effect on his life—but focused in one horrifying moment on Richard.

Soon after this episode it became increasingly clear that Richard was finding life less and less worth living. Richard spent an afternoon talking with one of the authors of this book. That evening Richard told Charles about the conversation, including his report of how grateful he was for Charles and Charles' loyalty to him. Charles responded to this revelation partly in anger and partly in fear: "Damn you! Why haven't you told me that you appreciate me?" Richard's reply was "Well, you know that I do." Charles replied, "Yes, I do, but I still need to hear that you do." Charles' sense of despair and inadequacy increased as Richard withdrew from him and others, sensing that his time to "go" was approaching.

Six weeks before Richard died Charles received a $10,000 bonus from work. They went out for dinner at a good restaurant. Their choice of restaurants was limited because none of Richard's suits fit him any longer. The evening went well except for Richard having some difficulty eating because of his poor eyesight and coordination. Charles enjoyed the evening, but the joy that usually accompanied the receipt of his annual bonus was missing. The $10,000 didn't mean anything this year. He realized that it couldn't keep Richard alive, take away Richard's pain, or remove the hurt that they both felt. Their relationship, cottage, futures were being destroyed by an insidious virus, and there was nothing Charles or anyone else could do about it.

Richard was unable to get out of bed the last four weeks of his life. Until this time they shared a bed, but Richard's incontinence made this no longer practical. He was placed in the guest bedroom while Charles stayed in their room. Weakened and blind, Richard lay in bed, dependent on Charles to feed, bathe, turn, and change him. Charles arose early to take care of Richard before he went to work. Two neighbors who remained loyal to Charles and Richard during the entire illness alternated coming in at noon to feed Richard and be company to him. Richard would then be alone until Charles came home, often as late as 8 or 9 P.M. They tried to talk, but there was little to say. Richard had decided to die. Charles respected his decision.

Apart from the two neighbors, Charles and Richard were alone during this final month. Charles worked each day but could not sleep at night. Two or three hours of restless sleep was the best that he could do. He paced, cried, worried, smoked cigarettes, and stared into a void while keeping an ear tuned to Richard's room for any sound indicating that Richard needed something. Charles became more fragile emotionally as Richard drew closer to death. The stress of AIDS was proving to be more than this twenty-six-year-old man could bear. He was bordering on a psychotic break when a man Richard had met at the clinic called to inquire about Richard. This stranger to Charles visited Richard and talked to Charles. A group of the stranger's friends organized to be with Richard and Charles during this final illness. Someone stayed with them every night, cooking, doing laundry, helping with Richard's care, talking to Charles. The first night someone stayed Charles ate a full meal and slept ten hours. Someone else in the house gave Charles security to sleep.

Charles stayed at home the last five days of Richard's life. He had to tell his boss and co-workers that his brother was dying in a distant city, lest they discover his homosexuality. He promised Richard that he would be there when he died. Charles kept his promise. While still holding Richard's lifeless body, he called the stranger to report that Richard had died and to ask him to return. Within minutes the stranger was there to assist Charles. The hospice nurse who was checking on Richard was summoned. The funeral directors with whom arrangements had been made for Richard's cremation were called. Richard had asked that expenses be kept to a minimum after he died. His body was to be cremated as soon as possible after his death. When his body left the home it was not to be seen again.

The hospice nurse suggested that Richard's body be dressed. She felt that it would be nicer for Charles to say good-bye to Richard if Richard were dressed in a suit, white shirt, and tie, rather than in a T shirt and diapers. Charles agreed. Clothes were selected. The hospice nurse and stranger gently prepared Richard's body, cleaning him, grooming him, dressing him, and positioning his body as it would be in a casket rather than in the fetal position in which he died. When these preparations were complete Charles said good-bye to Richard privately while the music and words of a popular song titled "Endless Love" echoed through the speakers that Richard had placed in every room.

Richard's illness and death cost Charles approximately $15,000. The financial burden was insignificant compared with the emotional cost. Charles does not regret being gay or loving Richard. He is frightened, however, about having another lover. The hurt accompanying Richard's illness and death was great. He does not want to be the survivor again. It hurts too much. Also, he is unsure how he will manage without Richard. He is afraid that he will not be strong enough to face his uncertain future. Charles thought that he would grow old with Richard. Now Richard is gone. Charles finds it difficult to make plans for the future. This isn't because he doesn't care about the future. It is because he has learned, at an early age, how vulnerable life is.

Like Richard, Charles is Roman Catholic. He prayed

frequently during their long ordeal. He asked God for strength, comfort, and guidance. He never tried to bargain with God for Richard's life or his own. Charles is not angry with God about AIDS or Richard's death. Neither event has lessened his faith in God. He thinks, however, that the churches could be more helpful in the AIDS crisis. No person, gay or straight, should face almost alone what he and Richard faced with AIDS. The churches and their leaders could fashion a more compassionate response if they will find the courage to do so. The close relationship that he and Richard enjoyed with a priest who took a personal interest in them is evidence to Charles that some Christians really do care. "Why," he asks, "can't the love of this one priest be expressed by all clergy and lay people?"

CHRIS

Chris and Todd were lovers. They met in a bar in February 1982. Chris was twenty-four years old; Todd was a year younger. It almost was love at first sight. They began to see each other once a week, then twice a week, then four times a week, and then, finally, every day. After ten weeks of being together, talking by phone, and exchanging cards and love notes, they decided to become lovers. Their first months together were Spartan. They had little money and no furniture for an apartment. They lived for three months with a friend who was renovating his house. Chris and Todd slept on blankets placed on the cold, wooden floor. The house was in a bad part of town. But despite this hardship, they were happy just to be together. The hard floor was made bearable as they lay together, holding each other, making plans for an apartment, furnishings, jobs, vacations, and other things that preoccupy young couples in love. They were alike in some ways and different in other ways. Chris was an extrovert, Todd was shy. Chris was impulsive, Todd was deliberate. Chris was wasteful, Todd was frugal. Chris was expressive, Todd was stoic. Their personality differences attracted them to each other as much as their mutual interests. They enjoyed television, movies, novels, car trips, pool, swimming, and eating out. They drank little alcohol and never used drugs recreationally. Each took pride in his appearance and their appearance as a couple. Chris was tall (6'6") and had dark hair and green eyes. Todd was shorter (5'10") and had brown hair and hazel eyes. They kept their bodies trim and strong by regular workouts in a gym.

Chris was from a rural community in Alabama. Todd came from a farming community in Indiana. Both were high school graduates, but neither attended college. They both had clerical jobs in financial firms. They enjoyed each other. As long as they had each other, a place to sleep, and food to eat, they thought they would be happy. They lived simply. They were in love and content. Then Todd went to a physician and their world began to change.

In April 1984 Todd was treated for a problem unrelated to AIDS. A series of blood tests indicated, however, that his immune response was compromised. The physician gave him news that sounds like a death sentence to gay men in the era of AIDS. Todd responded to the ominous news the same way that he responded to good news—matter-of-factly. He said little. Chris said much more. He rationalized that Todd's abnormal test results were explainable by something other than AIDS. He refused to accept that Todd might become ill. Todd was strong. He looked fit. He didn't have a fever, night sweats, diarrhea, fatigue, weight loss, or swollen glands. Without these warning signals, Chris thought, "Todd can't be coming down with AIDS."

A month later Todd became acutely ill. He was admitted to hospital and found to have an opportunistic infection in his brain. Chris could deny the truth no longer. Todd had AIDS. They were both afraid. Hospital rooms, brain biopsies, and intravenous treatments were new and frightening experiences for them. Chris told Todd, "We'll beat this. I'm going to take care of you. I'll make sure you eat right and rest a lot. This doesn't have to do to us what it's done to other people. I'm not going to desert you. You're not going to die." Todd recovered and went back to work as soon as he was able. This sequence of illness, hospitalization, and return to work was repeated five times between May 1984 and December 1985.

Chris' pledges of loyalty and perseverance were put to the test during Todd's illness. He was tempted to desert Todd on two occasions. The first time was in August 1984. Todd was very sick again. The magnitude of the disruption of Todd's illness to his life was becoming clearer. He asked himself why he didn't walk away from it all. Then Chris thought about what it would be like without Todd with him. Thoughts of running away were set aside. The second time he considered leaving was a year later. Todd was hospitalized again. The cycle of illness and recovery was wearing him down. Each illness evoked fear. Each recovery engendered hope. Chris was on an emotional roller coaster. He also became more concerned about his own health. His work and stress stemming from Todd's illnesses caused him to be fatigued. Chris worried about who would take care of him if he became ill. It was all Todd could do to take care of himself. When Todd got better, Chris thought, perhaps they should separate so that each of them could concentrate solely on taking care of himself.

As before, Chris could not leave Todd. Chris discovered, the more he thought, that he needed Todd, perhaps more than Todd needed him.

During the intervals between Todd's illnesses, they lived as normally as possible. They did not keep Todd's diagnosis a secret. A lesbian couple and a gay couple were their closest social friends. The six of them spent much time together. As Todd's illness progressed the four friends drifted away. Todd and Chris were basically left on their own. Neighbors stopped in periodically for brief visits and to inquire about Todd. More casual friends phoned. Todd felt badly that callers would ask Chris how Todd was feeling, rather than ask him directly when he answered the phone. Todd felt more comfortable talking about what was happening to him than they did. Todd didn't particularly want to talk about his illness with these people, he simply resented their inability or unwillingness to mention the subject to him.

Todd had a recurrence of the earlier brain infection in May 1985. He was successfully treated again and sent home. The infection, however, resulted in weakness on his right side and an involuntary tremor of his right arm and leg. Todd was unable to return to work. He was able to take care of himself at home. Household chores, reading, television, and videotape movies occupied his days when he was not visiting the clinic. During October, Todd grew weaker. He gradually became more dependent on Chris for his daily care. Chris began to do all the cooking, laundry, cleaning, and shopping, in addition to helping Todd with his medicines, bath, and toilet. The days grew longer for Chris as Todd grew weaker. Chris worked a full day and a full night. He phoned Todd six or eight times a day to see if he was all right. Each call ended with "I love you."

By the first week in November, Todd began to have a

fever. Diagnostic tests were negative at first. Weeks passed. Then a cough developed. His fever went higher. Chris and Todd had been through this before. They suspected that Todd was developing another lung infection that would require hospitalization. Todd was admitted to hospital on Friday morning.

Todd must have sensed that he was severely ill. He asked Chris the next day if he was going to make it. Chris, as always, was reassuring. Unfortunately, Chris was mistaken. By Sunday additonal drugs were given in an effort to control the lung infection. Todd's condition deteriorated rapidly. Oxygen was required. At 4 A.M. Monday morning Todd's parents, Ruth and David, were called. Chris remained at Todd's bedside. Ruth and David arrived Monday evening. They went directly to the hospital from the airport. They and Chris were told that Todd was in grave condition, that his survival was uncertain. (Ruth and David's story is told next in this chapter.)

Todd was terrified. He fought sleep. It seemed that he was afraid to sleep, fearing that he wouldn't awake. He was extremely weak and terrified on Tuesday. He was getting 100 percent oxygen. His breathing was labored and rapid. Speaking was almost impossible. He commented that it was a bright, sunny December day. Chris told him that it was ordered just for him. It was the last blue sky that Todd would see.

Throughout the day he fought sleep and tried to breathe. In exasperation he would say, "I can't breathe," and shake his head. His beautiful hazel eyes were filled with terror. Chris and Todd's parents did what they could to comfort him. A nurse's aide offered to rub Todd's back. With what little strength remained, Todd rolled on his side. The aide rubbed his fever-hot back for a few moments. Then, at the aide's suggestion, Chris, Todd's mother, and Todd's father took turns rubbing

Todd's back and speaking to him. After this he slept for a brief time. Still Todd's condition worsened. Another medication was proposed, even though the physicians doubted that it would save Todd's life. Todd told Chris that he "couldn't take any more." The additional drug was not started. Todd was sedated. Chris and Todd's parents stayed by Todd's side until he died at dawn on Wednesday morning at twenty-seven years of age.

Todd's body was cremated. Chris took the ashes to Indiana to attend a memorial service for Todd with Todd's family. On his return, Chris arranged for another memorial service in Houston. Christmas 1985 was not joyful for Chris. His lover of four years was dead. Chris was alone. A man who was weakened by AIDS paradoxically had been Chris' strength. Without Todd, without Todd's strength and courage, Chris felt lost. He realized that his love for Todd deepened as the months of Todd's illness passed. Chris realized that his attraction to Todd was more than physical or sexual. He learned that loving a person may require patience, understanding, and letting go. But mixed with his hurt and grief when Todd died, Chris felt anger. He was angry at AIDS, at Todd for dying, for leaving him. In Chris' words "How could he leave me? He knew how much I loved him and needed him. Todd often said that he couldn't take any more. I'd tell him not to give up. I need you, fight on! And without Todd saying a word, I could sense a renewed determination to get better. I think he fought so hard to live, even to the end, because he knew that I'd be lost without him. The hardest thing I've ever done in my life was to tell Todd OK, that he didn't have to fight any longer, after he said he couldn't take any more on Tuesday before he died." In short, Chris gave Todd permission to die.

From the beginning Chris repressed or denied the knowledge that Todd would die. He acknowledged this for the first time the day before Todd died. Todd never complained about anything. Just curling up together in bed to watch television was a special pleasure for the both of them after Todd became ill. Todd's increasing dependency, however, pained Chris. Todd was independent. He had his own mind. Becoming incontinent and wearing diapers was an indignity to Todd. Todd hated this and Chris hated it for him. Todd's helplessness was shared by Chris: "Watching someone you love work so hard to breathe and not be able to help is terrible. Looking into eyes that were begging for something to be done and not being able to help is terrible. But worst of all was seeing terror in his eyes and not being able to protect him or calm him." Chris got his strength from Todd, even as he neared death. Chris worries now if he will develop AIDS. Without having Todd for strength he doubts if he could face it.

Chris knew that even though he appeared to be more extroverted and decisive, Todd was his pillar of strength. The song that he chose for Todd's memorial service captures the true nature of their relationship. The lyrics to "Wind Beneath My Wings"[1] are the following:

> It must have been cold there
> In my shadow
> To never have sunlight on your face
> You've been content to let me shine
> You always walked a step behind
> I was the one with all the glory
> While you were the one with all the strength
> Only a face without a name
> And I never once heard you complain
> Did you ever know that you're my hero
> And everything I'd like to be
> I could fly higher than an eagle
> 'Cause you are the wind beneath my wings.

It might have appeared to go unnoticed
But I've got it all here in my heart
I want you to know I know the truth
I would be nothing without you.
Did you ever know that you're my hero
And everything I'd like to be
I could fly higher than an eagle
'Cause you are the wind beneath my wings
You are the wind beneath my wings.

Chris' grief was unrelenting. He felt that if he had loved Todd more, maybe he would not have died. He lamented that he should have done more to take care of Todd. If he had done more, Chris thought, maybe Todd would have lived until a cure is found. Chris constantly felt that he had not done enough, even though no one, including Todd, ever criticized him for not doing more. Chris was alone now. He could deceive himself no longer. The finality of Todd's death was most real to Chris at bedtime. Chris slept little and restlessly after Todd died. He would lie in bed remembering Todd, reliving Todd's final hospitalization, and cry for Todd and himself. One night between Christmas and New Year's when Chris could not sleep he decided to write down his feelings and thoughts. At 2 A.M. he wrote the following.

God, how I thought Todd was precious. At times he was like a little kid. He used to act like he was so much shorter than I and jump up in the air in order to reach to hit my shoulder. I couldn't say good-bye to my little friend the day he died and I can't say good-bye now. He was so cute. I'd ask him to sing me a love song and what he'd do was he'd make up syllables that made no sense whatsoever and sing them as off key as his vocal cords would manage and we would hold each other and laugh as if we would never let go of each other because I knew that it was in fact love songs he serenaded me with, only he and I were the only persons on earth that understood what it was he was singing. I always thought we'd be together forever. I used to think 1986 would find a cure or at least a satisfactory treatment that would have been beneficial to Todd, but now I look to 1986 with complete dread. Not only do I not know what 1986 may hold in store for me, health or otherwise, I must face it alone and without Todd. As I've said many times over, Todd was my only source of strength and courage. Now I'm scared to death. All that I've known for the past four years was Todd. We loved each other so very much. We didn't need kinky sex or a college degree or anything. All we ever needed or wanted was each other. But the time we had together was short, so mercilessly short. We'd just begun to grow together. Once Todd was taken to Brennan's [an exclusive restaurant] for his birthday and that for him was a wonderful and very special event. We always talked of going to Brennan's. Something special like our anniversary. Todd just wanted to share that specialness with me. We never went. I can just see the smile on his face and his beautiful eyes in the candlelight of Brennan's. We talked of going camping in Austin. The January after Todd was diagnosed we bought a tent on sale and planned on going in the springtime. We thought there would be time for all that. But now he is gone and we will never do any of the things we wanted to share together. We'll never take baths together, or midnight swims, evening walks in the summertime. I'll never hold Todd again. No more touching and holding him and running my fingers through his hair. I *need* to touch and hold him tonight. I want to explode because this feeling is so overwhelming. I can't hold him and I won't explode. There is no other way to describe how I feel right now. Todd needed to be held by me and I needed to hold him. I need to hold him now but he's gone. I can't touch a memory. They are intangible. They are not solid. They do absolutely nothing to satisfy the physical need. All memories do is make me sad, memories of Todd's smile and memories of his eyes, those beautiful eyes, and his hair. Memories of him saying how much he loved me, the way he'd say it. And when I'd tell him I love him, he'd look at me with those beautiful eyes and say, oh poof, I know you do. Memories of how he smiled when he'd say that. Memories of all the love in that smile and in his heart, and in his eyes. All of these wonderful memories of Todd are just the things that make the need to touch him tonight so overwhelming. Todd was so special to me, my little angel in heaven, and the love I feel for him so dear. I only hope that there was no doubt in his mind of that when he died. There were times when the stress of Todd's illness got the best of me. But that never lessened my love for him ever. He went away too soon. I have so much more inside to give him. All that is inside me right now Todd gave to me. He gave me extraordinary strength and courage. He gave to me love and understanding and compassion. Because of Todd everything I do, see, touch has a new meaning. I see all of Todd's gentleness in sunshine, or clouds, children, flowers, puppies, rain. He is in everything around me. I see in everything all the beauty and gentleness that made up Todd's being. No one will ever know just how Todd has made this world a better place for me. My sweet and gentle Todd. I love and miss you so much. If only I could touch you again.

Chris continues to work through his grief. Support from his family, friends, and co-workers has been helpful. Phone calls and letters from Todd's family expressing concern for him also have helped him to feel that he is not alone and abandoned. Chris also has called on his faith for strength and comfort. He is not angry at God for what has happened. To the contrary, he thanks God in prayer for letting him and Todd be together for four years. Chris thinks that Todd enriched and changed his life. He feels that his relationship with Todd and their struggle together with AIDS have taught him how to love more purely, to be understanding and patient, to be more compassionate and sensitive, and to be less selfish. Without Todd and his fight to live, Chris doubts that he would have learned certain lessons about life, including the place of character and virtue in it. The gentleness, perseverance, and courage that Todd exhibited in his battle with disease and death are now examples for Chris to emulate in his effort to live without the "wind beneath my wings."

RUTH AND DAVID

Ruth and David are the parents of Todd, whose story partly was incorporated into the story about Chris. David was working at a small manufacturing plant in Indiana when he married Ruth. Todd was their second child, but their first son. They enjoyed being parents and loved children. Three more children followed Todd, two sons and one daughter. They remember that Todd displayed the same character traits as a child that he did as an adult. He was well behaved, courteous, gentle, self-reliant, and concerned about others. Todd enjoyed being with his grandparents and other elderly people. Often he would go to the county home for the elderly to visit the residents. He enjoyed hearing the stories they would tell about their younger years, their experiences on the farms, travels, and life during "the wars."

Todd also enjoyed plants as a youth, especially those that bloomed. He often made arrangements of flowers from the yard to give to his mother. She frequently received live plants from Todd as gifts on special occasions. Ruth cherished them all, and the plants that are still alive are even more special now that Todd is gone.

Todd had an interest in music as a child. David and Ruth bought him a small organ to test his talent. He had a good ear, learning how to play on his own. A larger organ replaced the smaller one as a gift on his thirteenth birthday. Todd loved to play, often playing late at night. He sang as he played. As might be expected in a home where the church was an important part, Todd sang in the choir when he became old enough. At times, he played organ for Sunday worship.

Todd enjoyed being with his siblings and friends. He didn't date much as a teenager. Ruth and David never gave this much thought. There was one girl whom Todd seemed to like. Both had an interest in music. But on the whole, Todd only had dates with girls to attend special events at the rural high school.

After finishing high school Todd went to a nearby city to work for one year. Then he returned home to work. But after another year he seemed dissatisfied with life in a small town. He began to travel each night to the small city nearby. Then Todd elected to move to the small city, where he lived with a roommate. David and Ruth did not suspect at the time that Todd's roommate was a boyfriend. In retrospect, however, they now understand their relationship, since Todd moved to Houston because his roommate did. Todd took a new roommate after settling in Houston—Chris. Ruth and David didn't like Todd being so far away from home. They thought that it would be inappropriate to object too strongly. He was on his own and should be free to make his own decisions.

David and Ruth kept in contact with Todd when he was away from home. Todd would be at home for holidays and special occasions. The family members were close to one another even though the children went their separate ways after graduating from high school.

Todd went home for a visit in July 1984. He did not tell them that he had been ill. Neither did he tell them that he was gay. David and Ruth thought that he looked thin and did not appear at ease around them. Ruth, as mothers tend to do, thought that Todd was not eating well. Ruth and David attributed his behavior to his preference to be on his own rather than being at home with Mom and Dad. His visit went well. Todd said nothing about what was happening to him. He never complained about anything. He tended to keep to himself information that he thought would upset others.

David and Ruth independently speculated that Todd was homosexual soon after he finished school. They never spoke to each other about their suspicions. Todd's life-style and interests were rationalized to be due to something other than being homosexual. His brothers and sisters also suspected Todd's sexuality. But, like their parents, they said nothing to one another or their mom and dad. By not speaking the word or voicing the question they all thought that maybe their suspicions were unfounded.

After Todd's move to Texas his letters home began to refer to "Chris and I" or "we." No one wanted to believe that Todd was gay, but by now all of the family were reasonably sure. Despite their conviction no one treated Todd differently than they treated one another. His life-style was never a topic of discussion or an impediment to their love. David and Ruth did not have their suspicions confirmed until they arrived in Houston to be with him when he died. Facing this truth created an additional and different sort of sadness, at this time, than the grief and concern they felt on learning that Todd was near death. David and Ruth do not know why Todd was gay. Had they known earlier, they now speculate, perhaps Todd could have helped them to understand. Nevertheless, an earlier awareness would not have caused them not to love Todd, or to reject him.

Ruth and David gradually learned that Todd was severely ill. Todd minimized his illnesses to them at first. He assured them that he was getting better, that he would be fine. However, the frequency of his illnesses and the hospitalizations caused David and Ruth to think that he was more seriously ill than they had been told. Both Todd and Chris seemed to avoid the subject whenever possible. Ruth thought several times about asking a lot of questions. But when they talked by phone, Todd always seemed able to keep the conversation on other topics. As with Todd's homosexuality, Ruth and David learned that Todd had AIDS and that Chris was his lover when they arrived in Houston for the last time. Ruth and David, again independently and never talking together about it, wondered in July 1985 if Todd had AIDS. He visited home for a week. He didn't want to do anything strenuous. He was still weakened from a recent hospitalization. Everything he used had to be sterile. He regularly took his temperature. His medicines were taken on schedule, including liquid medicines that he injected into an indwelling catheter.

This was Todd's last visit home. Everyone had a good time together. The family played cards and board games together at night. During the days Todd went to movies, visited old friends, or spent time with his grandparents. After Todd returned to Houston, Ruth and David secretly thought that Todd looked less healthy and even thinner than when he visited a year earlier. Todd said nothing to alarm them. They asked nothing that might have upset his visit. But silently they wondered if their fears could be true.

David and Ruth's faith was important to them as they came to know the truth about Todd. Their conservative Christian beliefs do not approve of homosexuality. But despite these negative judgments David and Ruth loved Todd when they only thought that he was gay and when they knew for certain. In their words, "We sure didn't approve of Todd's relationship with Chris, but he was still our son and we still loved him. We wouldn't have turned him or Chris away knowing of his life-style or illness. We believe all people have sinned and we cannot say one is more sinful than another. We don't believe God sent AIDS on gay people or on Todd. Good church-going people die of cancer. Do we say God sent it on them? No. Neither has God sent AIDS as a punishment."

Even though David and Ruth never wavered in their love for Todd or their faith in God during this traumatic time, they told no one outside the family the truth about Todd or his illness. It was difficult at times to know how to answer church friends who would ask what was wrong with Todd or how he was doing. David and Ruth asked the church to pray for Todd. They prayed themselves. In their words, "We learned how much it helps to have a God that we can tell everything. At times we would fall asleep praying and crying. We believed that we were not alone, that God was with us and Todd, and that he loved us all. This made it a little easier to bear."

David and Ruth told their pastor about Todd as the memorial service was being planned. He issued no judgments and provided them with pastoral support. Most of the congregation attended the service. Food was brought to the family home. Flowers, cards, and personal words conveyed the sympathy and love of their Christian friends. Chris and a friend who accompanied him to attend the service were introduced to everyone as Todd's roommate and friend, respectively. No one asked a question.

David and Ruth's experience has brought them closer to God and their church. They found that, with God's help, they could get through a crisis that they never thought they could. They still don't fully understand why one of their five children was homosexual. Neither do they understand why the AIDS virus appeared.

They know something about the power of parental and divine love. It was these types of love, and the love they saw that Todd and Chris had for each other, that sustained them when it seemed that they could bear no more hurt and pain. It has even enabled them to reach out to Chris out of concern for him in his grief. They and Todd's brothers and sisters treated him as one of the family while he was there for Todd's memorial service. Ruth has phoned him several times in the months since Todd died to see how he is doing. Even Todd's grandmother has maintained contact with him. This small, wrinkled, white-haired, rural lady in her seventies sent the following letter to Chris after he attended Todd's memorial service.

Dear Chris:

We have lots more snow up here and it's cold! Went over to the bank, and to the post office for stamps and my big long coat sure felt good. Hope you and Greg [a friend who went with Chris] had a good trip back. We are all so glad you could come. It meant a lot to meet Todd's best friend and another friend, to know that he had such a good life during his short stay on earth until he got so bad sick. And he always seemed to have a cheerful hope even then. Which only we Christians can really have.

I asked him if you were a Christian, Chris. He never did get around to telling me. I hope so—you certainly have the qualities to be a good one. Grandpa and I both noticed how like Todd you are in so many ways. Tho, of course not in looks, ha! We will miss Todd until we can meet him again. But how we treasure having had him as long as we did. I'm sure heaven is happier because he has come. Please tell your parents how much we appreciate their loving kindness to Todd. Todd loved to visit them with you and all his friends who have shared in his care—and helped him so much to endure what he had to go through. When we couldn't be there—God did supply his every need. God always does. I hope you will read and enjoy the devotion book *Streams in the Desert* that I gave Todd this summer. It meant a lot to me to have him have it.

I hope you get to go to your parents for the holidays. And remember, God knows we have sad hearts and he will comfort us—by reminding us of the joy and peace he sent the world through his son. The son who saves all who believe and are baptized into Jesus Christ for the remission of sins. For those who keep the faith, will come Eternal life.

That is why we are here, to prepare ourselves. So our task is to continue that preparation until our time comes to depart. Then we'll see Todd again.

God bless you.

Todd's grandma

write.

David, Ruth and their family are comforted by God's love for them, Todd and Chris. Their ability to respond in a redemptive fashion to disclosures and events that were hurtful grew out of a belief in the sufficiency of love. Their love for Todd, one another, and God was translated into a love for Chris, who had become part of them through his love and commitment to Todd. They embodied and expressed in their response to Todd's lifestyle, illness, and death the instruction of Paul to the church at Corinth regarding the gift of love. Paul's words were their guide: "Love is patient and kind. . . . Love does not insist on its own way. . . . Love bears all things, believes all things, hopes all things, endures all things. Love never ends. . . . So faith, hope, love abide, these three; but the greatest of these is love [1 Cor. 13:4–5, 7–8, 13]."

136

SARAH AND MARK

Charles was born into a close and loving family in which the values of family togetherness provided the foundation out of which other values and attitudes were formed. His two older sisters vied to care for him as a baby, and even in later years, when young brothers can so easily offend older sisters, he seemed able to do no wrong in their eyes. It was all the more painful to Sarah and Mark when, at twenty-one, Charles arrived home at their south Texas ranch to tell them that he was gay and that he had AIDS. The double shock left them bewildered and in deep pain. At first they seemed unsure as to which hurt was the deepest. After the initial crisis they sought to understand from Charles the answers to the questions: "Why . . .?" "How . . .?" They resolved most of the distress by deciding together that, in the face of the constantly recurring infections and lesions, they would take only one course of action. With his agreement they moved his belongings from his city apartment to their home and began caring for him. In the course of their conversations they learned that Charles had discussed his situation with his sisters and their husbands, and that the children had agreed that their parents would only be hurt deeply if they learned that their son was gay. It was only when he contracted AIDS that the "secret" could be kept no longer.

Charles was a gifted young man, interested in music and sports. His greatest gift, however, was his warm, loving personality. Sarah and Mark were somewhat overwhelmed, both during the funeral and subsequently, by the flood of letters and messages they received from people who had known Charles. One of their most poignant memories is of one of his junior high school teachers, who shared with them, through her tears, incidents she remembered from his school days. People whom they had never met told them stories that indicated the extent of Charles' influence on them, including an incident recounted by a family for which he had been a baby-sitter. They knew he had made no enemies unless there were some who envied his giving and loving nature. He was respected by those who knew him. Each story confirmed their own perceptions of Charles as a person of integrity in whom the values by which they had lived were manifested. Proud as they were to learn so much from his circle of friends, they could not forget that he had excluded them from part of his life. That he had made his decision out of love for them, seeking to protect them from hurt, somehow only made the hurt deeper.

During the times when they accompanied Charles on hospital visits, often to the outpatient clinic for treatments, they met other families whose stories were so like their own that they were often taken aback by the similarity. Family after family had decided not to share their sons' illness with their pastors or the members of their parishes. They began to envy those parents who were able to turn to clergy and congregations for support, but they were so few. Sarah could remember sitting in that awful waiting area, with no sense of privacy, but where, finding that the woman sitting near her was there for the same reason as herself, they shared their tears and despair. Sarah and Mark had joined their present parish only two years before Charles' return home and, for that reason, chose not to divulge their pain or its source to their priest. Perhaps they misjudged him, Sarah sometimes thought, but the risk of misunderstanding or rejection seemed greater than the benefits of such a disclosure. During the period of three months in which Charles lived with them before his death, they experienced a great deal of support from both pastor and members. Although they did not have a strong relationship within the congregation, it became known that Charles was ill. They described his medical problem as cancer, which accounted for his continuing pneumonia and lesions. Their immediate neighbors have been particularly sensitive to their grief since Charles' death, inviting them to share in community activities. A recent fund-raiser for the American Cancer Society was a point at which they could begin to reenter local community functions, although it also brought back sad memories.

Still the questions remain. Why Charles? Why us? He never did anything to harm anyone. Why our son? Sarah and Mark cannot find answers to their questions and are becoming aware that they may never do so. At least they have never thought of his illness as a punishment, and they cannot blame God for what happened. If you were able to speak with parents of other people with AIDS, they were asked, what would you want to say to them? Their answer was simple and direct: "Whatever you do, stand by your children. Do not shun them. Let your children know you love them."

JOAN AND FRED

Joan and Fred were known to friends in the neighborhood as "a typical happily married couple." Their two children, David and Beth, were attractive, well-liked youngsters. The family possessed all the characteristics of middle-class America: good health, two cars, pleasant home, and stable income from secure professional employment, Fred as an industrial engineer, Joan as a junior college instructor. Joan left the college faculty when the children were young. When Beth, the

139

younger child, reached the age of five, Joan began to teach part-time. In 1975 Fred collapsed at work and died three days later. There were no warnings of heart problems. As Joan put it later, she was unprepared for widowhood. She returned to teaching full time in order to see David and Beth through college. That goal was reached in 1985. She began to feel securer. Tulsa was feeling the impact of the crisis in the petrochemical industries, but her own position seemed assured.

In May 1985, while visiting David in Dallas, her world collapsed again. David informed her that he had been diagnosed with AIDS, and that he had accepted his homosexuality in 1980. Stunned by the disclosures, she did not remain immobilized for long. She flew home to complete necessary business arrangements and then returned to Dallas, where she found an apartment and settled into the weekly routine of clinic visits and chemotherapy treatments. David moved in with his mother. Fortunately, his general health was good, and he seldom missed a full day of work. But now his work place was the family apartment. He was graduated as a design engineer with a glowing academic record and was sought by a number of companies. He joined a large firm of industrial architects and received a series of rapid promotions. Two weeks prior to being diagnosed with AIDS, he received his most recent promotion as a full member of the staff. He was aware that his immediate supervisor was also gay, although that was not known within the firm. David informed his supervisor of his situation, and three days later he was informed that he had been placed on medical leave with full pay. When he protested he was told that this action was to protect other employees from contracting AIDS. David pointed out that all the available medical information indicated that this was not a risk. Nevertheless, the restriction remained in force. He was faced with the decision either to accept his status or to contest the firm's action on grounds of discrimination. Resigning his position was ruled out. He consulted an attorney, only to find that he had no grounds for a legal complaint. On the surface the firm's action was generous and had broken no laws. David felt that he was in a no-win situation.

It became clear to David that the firm was refusing to permit him to visit the office because of the senior staff's fear of losing clients if his medical status became known. He was humiliated when, soon after he contracted AIDS, he went to the building but was forced to remain at the front door. A staff member gave him verbal instructions through the closed door. Another reason for the firm's actions then emerged. David was accompanied by his attorney when the final arrangements for his continuing employment were negotiated. The possibility that he would seek damages for wrongful dismissal was indicated. It then became known that one of the firm's principals was planning to stand for elective office. He feared the consequences to his political hopes if David was dismissed and the firm became involved in a highly publicized legal action for damages.

David's most serious problem was not the catastrophic impact of the AIDS virus; for the moment, his medical problems were minimal. The mental and emotional impact was much greater. His work at the firm had been meticulous, always above average in quality. He drove himself with a goal of perfection that made his work invaluable to the company. His application to the highest professional standards was reflected in the neatness of his dress. David's supervisors always praised his commitment to the firm's interests. Being isolated from his work team and forced to work in the office he furnished at home, David was denied the conditions in which he did his best work: as a peer working in close relationship with his associates. He now wore jeans to work in the next room instead of the pin-striped suit as was his custom. Moreover, the indignity and sense of injustice evoked by the firm's actions left him frustrated and angry, hardly conditions in which he could continue to produce at the level he expected of himself. He received his assignments in packages left by messengers at the apartment door! There were few consolations, but those he did receive were essential to his ability to work. Joan affirmed her love for her son, as did his sister, Beth. Despite the firm's insistence that they were merely protecting his fellow employees, many of his co-workers visited on the way home from work or during weekends and shared with David the frustration now imposed on him.

Joan felt his hurt and frustration keenly. Her own anger now focused not only on the firm, but also on people in her denomination who linked AIDS with God's punishment on people who suffer AIDS. She began to look for opportunities to bring such issues to the public's attention but felt alone and vulnerable. Furthermore, if she took any public stand, her action might endanger David's tenuous relationship with his company, and he needed that security for the continuation of income and medical benefits. Her needs were partly met in a parents' support group, but her anguish was sharpened as she learned how other AIDS patients and their families have fared. She learned, for example, that Robert's job had been terminated by his company, forcing him to change his employer's insurance coverage to an individual policy at a crippling cost. A group of people with AIDS, she found, had been provided accommodation in a hostel. But because they were too ill to maintain full employment, they spent time in idleness, watching daytime TV. Many of them became depressed. After visiting them she feared for what might have happened to David had she not been able to assist him.

The cost of moving to Dallas was high for Joan, although she did not hesitate to respond to David's need. But the loss of her job means that she is forced to withdraw savings to meet living expenses. Although she is not immediately threatened financially, her anxiety is rising. She is unable to find a teaching position. She is seeking other types of employment but is finding that in the present depressed economy, her options are limited. A lifelong church member, she is distressed by indications that few church people and denominational officers seem ready to bring the needs of AIDS patients or their families to the attention of the general public. She is not sure what she expects in terms of specific actions, but she knows that most people do not want to be with people who have AIDS and are reluctant to be identified in any way with the care of those who have the disease. She had expected more from people of faith. If the church does not respond to this need, is there any other group that can be expected to do so?

Nurses,
Social Workers,
and Physicians

5

CINDY

Cindy has been a registered nurse for ten years. She began to see patients with AIDS in surgery in 1982. Stories about how some personnel, from physicians to housekeepers, were afraid to serve this population began to circulate in the hospital. She could not understand this discriminatory response. She became increasingly aware that, because of their fears or their dislike for AIDS patients, many of her peers either refused to care for them or provided less competent and compassionate care than they should. As a result, she requested a transfer from surgery to the outpatient clinic where people with AIDS and ARC are followed.

Her work in the clinic quickly shaped her views about AIDS and the people who suffer with this disease. She no longer saw people with AIDS as a group. Rather, as she got to know the patients they became individuals, unique, unlike one another except for their common struggle against a deadly virus. Their disease, sexuality, and life-style, she discovered, were stigmas that resulted in their not receiving the same sympathy, compassion, understanding, and support that is provided to almost any person with a fatal disease. Instead, people with AIDS are told that they deserve it. Commercial nursing home and inpatient hospice care are denied to them. Insurance benefits may be denied on the putative basis that their acute illnesses are preexisting conditions. Jobs are at times taken from them. Families, friends, and lovers sometimes leave them to care for themselves as best they can and die alone. That some of the patients experience one or more of these losses contributes to Cindy's sense of special responsibility to them, both professionally and personally.

Cindy also is drawn to people with AIDS because they are physically fragile and can be emotionally fragile. The course of the disease can be unpredictable. A patient can look reasonably good on Friday, with no acute illness, and Monday be hospitalized and by Wednesday, die. Because people with AIDS tend to know how vulnerable they are to infection and death, they seem to live in fear. Cindy tries to be optimistic and hopeful for each one. She tries to treat them, as nearly as possible, as if they were "normal." A result of her approach is that she gets to know many of the patients' histories, stories, personalities, moods, feelings, and idiosyncrasies. In short, they are persons to whom she can—and often does—become attached. Seeing these special people deteriorate and die causes her grief. And because there are so many patients and their deaths come at such close intervals, Cindy experiences chronic grief. She doesn't get to work through her grief properly before the cycle starts again. It is easier for her to accept the death of a patient who is ready to die. But when they fight hard to live and can't, their deaths anger her. In her words, "When they're not ready, I'm not ready."

Cindy considers it a privilege to work with this population. In her mind, to stereotype gay men with AIDS as "gutter sluts" is unfair. She admits that some have lived "fast and free," but by far these predominantly young adults are responsible and hardworking. Some are par-

145

ents, some are part of a couple, and others are alone. But almost without exception, Cindy sees them individually and corporately as people of courage, humor, charm, wit, and a limitless variety of interests. She is impressed by the care and concern that they show for one another, especially the support that the longer-term patients provide for those who are newly diagnosed. These long-term patients are inspirations for the others. When one dies, hope tends to fade temporarily for the rest.

Cindy has been impressed with the dedication of friends to people with AIDS. She acknowledges angrily that some friends and lovers have fled the scene. But she admires the friends who stick with a patient for weeks or months. Further, she wishes that more people could observe the strength of the love shared by homosexual lovers. Her ability to share life and death with people who are shunned by the majority is quite satisfying. For her, sharing small victories—big victories are not presently possible—and being appreciated for what she does are major professional and personal rewards.

Homosexuality and bisexuality have never been issues for Cindy. She thinks that prejudice and ignorance about sexuality have contributed to the abuse and neglect that people with AIDS have experienced from government, the public, and health care personnel. The effect of prejudice and ignorance on patients is frustrating to Cindy. She thinks that people with AIDS should concentrate on their disease and care, rather than preoccupy themselves with fighting for their rights. They should be respected as persons and be allowed to die with dignity. Cindy also is frustrated by the current inability of medicine to cure AIDS. At times she thinks that things are getting better. But then she realizes that the total number of patients that she sees is growing, even though patients are dying all the time. Further, Cindy is concerned for families of patients who cannot grieve properly because they are afraid to tell the people in their normal support groups what they are experiencing. AIDS, according to Cindy, destroys more than cells and immune systems in patients.

Cindy is divorced, with a teenaged son and daughter. They, and the remainder of her family, know of her work. Their reaction initially focused on her safety. They wanted her to be careful. When everyone was satisfied that she was safe, their hesitations were removed. In fact, her children seem proud of her and her work with people who are ostracized by others. As far as Cindy knows, her children's friends have not withdrawn from them. Her son and daughter have gotten to know some of the patients when they have been in Cindy's home. The children, like Cindy, have grown to see them for who they are: people with problems, often with no one to help and no place to go. Even so, they seem to care for her as a person. They ask how she is, take her to lunch, and minister to her when they sense that she is stressed.

Everything in the clinic isn't doom and gloom. The patients bring humor where the activity is deadly serious. One gay patient, who is quite personable, one morning put on a wig and makeup. He inflated rubber gloves and stuffed them inside his shirt, to simulate breasts. Then he ran into the clinic waiting area screaming, "I went to give blood and look what they did to me!" On another occasion three patients were talking about people they knew. Two of the three were trying to convince the third that he surely knew someone. After thinking for a time he responded in an exaggerated, campy fashion, "Oh, I may not remember him, but I'm sure I've had him!" Unfortunately, too often the laughter turns into a somber silence when a patient who is visibly near death arrives in a wheelchair or on a stretcher.

Cindy was brought up in the Roman Catholic Church, but she left it twenty years ago. Her work with patients who are dying with AIDS awakened her sense of need for God. She observed that the patients who were at peace with God seemed to have a better attitude about life and approached death peacefully. Now she attends a nondenominational Christian fellowship that positively values people regardless of their gender or sexuality. Cindy has no patience with clergy or churches that claim AIDS is God's punishment on homosexual men. Her God is loving, accepting, caring, and forgiving. She thinks that the people who say they worship this kind of God should not reject people with AIDS or ARC. They should offer spiritual, physical, and emotional support ministries. Then she thinks that they will be practicing what they preach. She is encouraged by the ministries some churches are beginning to provide.

Cindy soberly acknowledges that the treatment of AIDS complications only prolongs the inevitable. She tries to be optimistic to patients about news reports of experimental drugs that appear promising. In her heart, however, she sees little hope for patients within the next five years. In the interim, she expects her grief to be compounded but looks forward to the day when, in her words, "I can go look at the stars on a clear night and exclaim—guys, we did it! It's been worth it!"

DOROTHY

Like Cindy, Dorothy works in an outpatient clinic. She has been a registered nurse for four years. Since April 1985 Dorothy has worked with AIDS patients only as outpatients. Before then she worked with hospitalized AIDS patients, seeing them in all stages of the disease. Dorothy has never been afraid of catching AIDS from her patients. Her physician wanted her to change jobs while she was pregnant. She discussed the matter with her husband, who does not work in medicine. They decided that the risks to her and the pregnancy were insignificant. Dorothy continues to care for people with AIDS. She chose to care for them initially. Her commitment strengthens as time passes.

Dorothy shares many observations and concerns with Cindy. Unlike Cindy, Dorothy is an active member in a Protestant church that condemns homosexuality. At first she thought that AIDS was God's punishment on people, not just gay men, for their excesses. These thoughts soon were questioned as she came to know the patients. They were people who, in the main, did not fit the stereotype of gay men—narcissistic, hedonistic, offensive. If their sexuality or life-style is sinful, in her mind, it is no greater sin than any other type. She had been taught that God loves and forgives and wants people to love and forgive. Thus, Dorothy now thinks that homosexual acts may be sinful; but loving, even if it is for a person of the same sex, can never be sinful.

Dorothy considers nearly all her patients to be "nice" people. Through them she now understands what it is like to be victimized, abandoned, powerless, subject to discrimination. She and her husband advocate gay rights and support "gay causes." She isn't shocked by their personal histories. She is, however, shocked by the way some of the patients have been treated by family or friends. For example, she feels a special sympathy for one patient who was fired when his boss discovered that he had AIDS. His job paid little. He had no reserves. He wanted to go home but his parents said no. He didn't want to be an imposition on his friends. He gathered his

149

few possessions, put them in his car, and lived in his car for weeks.

She tries to understand her patients' fears. They have reasons to be afraid. Even she is shocked at times by the rapid changes they experience, from being reasonably well to being nearly totally dependent. She marvels at the hope and optimism she sees. Cancer patients, for example, reasonably can have hope. Chemotherapies can put their disease into remission. People with AIDS tend only to deteriorate and die, some quickly and others more slowly. Maybe a cure will come soon. In the meantime Dorothy wants to do her best to treat her patients decently and with respect.

Dorothy's grief for her patients is not limited to their deaths. It is especially painful for her to see patients who have neurological complications. They know that "they are losing it." Their frustration and anger about losing these capabilities seem more intense than their reaction to weight loss or visible cancer lesions. In her words, "People in their twenties and thirties just aren't supposed to be senile." Independence and self-determination are important to the patients. Dorothy thinks that they feel dehumanized and like infants when their neurological and physical losses are so severe that they become almost or totally dependent. Their grief over this abrupt change becomes a source of grief for her.

People with AIDS have educated Dorothy. She has learned about differences among people, life-styles, and values. She has been challenged intellectually, emotionally, and spiritually. Dorothy wishes that people, including people of faith, could set aside their prejudices and preconceptions about people with AIDS long enough to understand how often such people are mistreated and how much they suffer. Then perhaps the education she has been privileged to receive could be had by others. And in the end, people with AIDS would be treated decently and with the respect that they deserve.

JANET

Janet is a veteran nurse. She has practiced nursing for nearly thirty years. Now she is head nurse on a unit where people with AIDS receive in-hospital care. She has worked with AIDS patients since there have been AIDS patients.

In 1981, when people with AIDS were admitted to her floor, Janet was struck by how quickly they became ill, deteriorated, and died. The rapidity with which they died was in stark contrast to her experience with cancer patients, who would be acutely ill, receive treatment, and be in remission for an extended time before experiencing another acute episode or dying. The relentless, debilitating effect of AIDS was mysterious and frightening to her.

Janet was concerned for her patients who were reeling from life-threatening infections, for her staff, and for other patients on the floor whose immune status was depressed after chemotherapy for cancer. The nature of the risks associated with the care of this population and their magnitude were not known at this time. The anxiety of her staff was appreciably high. Infection control procedures were adopted and these anxieties abated. Unfortunately, the number of patients did not abate. Soon it became obvious that this disease was not going to disappear in six months. Janet and her staff geared up for the long haul.

The patients who were admitted in the early days were almost exclusively gay men. Many had lived in the fast lane. Their histories of numerous sex partners, drug use, and sexual practices, contained in the charts, were an offense to some of the nursing staff. In addition, some of the slang terms and descriptions of sexual activities were shocking. Finally, the appearance, conversation, and behavior of some visitors were upsetting. Nevertheless, the staff endeavored to provide competent, sensitive nursing care. No one ever said that these patients deserved what was happening to them. The general impression was that no one, regardless of who they were or what they had done, deserved to have this many severe illnesses and die such a terrible death.

The nurses received a crash course in alternate lifestyles. One man who operated a gay escort service continued to work from his hospital room. Symbols of sexual preference and body ornaments were surprising. Even though these sights shocked some staff, they were no more shocking than the way some patients were rejected and abandoned by family, lover, and friends. Janet remembers a twenty-four-year-old man who was kicked out by his lover, deserted by his family, and fired by his boss. He had no place to go when he was well enough to be discharged. Finally, after staying in the hospital for a week longer than necessary, his grandmother reluctantly agreed to take him. She also remembers a father who arrived two to three weeks before his son died. The father made arrangements for the disposition of his son's body and then left. The nurses were told not to bother to call him when his son died.

The early patients, in Janet's memory, tended to be exhibitionistic, demanding, and narcissistic. Part of their assertiveness may have been due to neurological complications that were not understood at the time. Now the description of the patients that she sees has changed. Although still predominantly young gay men, they tend not to be fast-lane people. Many are in relationships of several years' length. Lovers are deserting them less frequently. Families are present more. Fewer patients are requesting that families not be told of their sexuality or diagnosis. Perhaps some of the stigma of AIDS is lessening, perhaps not. Horror stories are still heard.

Caring for AIDS patients is different from caring for other patients with a chronic or terminal illness. People with AIDS often have several major illnesses at once, requiring multiple treatment protocols and an increased amount of staff time to implement them. The infection control procedures of gloves, mask, and gown consume valuable time and delay answering calls for service. AIDS patients tend to stay hospitalized longer. Staff get to know them and like them. Their deaths, as a result, are much harder to accept. Like Cindy, Janet and her nurses experience chronic grief. For example, during December 1985 thirteen patients on Janet's floor died of AIDS. These deaths were in addition to the normal death rate associated with the other thirty patients on her floor.

AIDS patients tend to require more emotional support than do other patients. They are young and see themselves as dying. They may be afraid, distrustful, and angry. They may sense, accurately, that some physicians resent having to care for them. (Some physicians are nice to gay patients in their presence and then call them names outside the room.) Patients often desire information that is not known. They may seek assurances that cannot be given. The emotional drain on patients and nursing staff can be severe. The stresses can increase when decisions are required and the patient is unable to make them. For example, who is the next of kin legally authorized to act—divorced spouse, child, parent, sibling? No one may be available, and when someone is contacted they may decline to act. In the meantime the patient "hangs over the abyss" and the medical and nursing staff are less certain about what to do. As time passed, the AIDS population, with all its variety, came to be seen by Janet as people who suffer and who may deserve preferential care because of the injustices done to them elsewhere.

Janet's work with people with AIDS has enabled her, and nearly all her staff, to become more understanding and sympathetic toward gay and bisexual men. Janet thinks that others ought not to make gay people suffer because of who they are. AIDS is burden enough. Intravenous drug abusers, however, are seen differently. Janet thinks that they have more of a choice about the risks they run. Further, they introduce or recruit others to abuse drugs. Homosexual people, in her judgment, do not choose their sexuality or convert people from heterosexual to homosexual.

Janet's staff consists mainly of young adults who identify with young patients. They have chosen to work on her unit. Many stay for a long time, others transfer quickly because the stress, work load, and grief become overwhelming. But for the staff who stay, like Janet, working with people who have AIDS has become a satisfying experience. Many of the patients, in her words, "worm their way into your heart." They are kind, appreciative, and try to minimize the number of times they call for help. The love, care, and devotion of some lovers have become an inspiration. For Janet, most of the patients are decent people who ought to be treated with respect and be allowed to die with dignity. The staff tends to invest themselves in patients who have repeated admissions. The patients' lovers, families, and friends become familiar. And when a patient is alone the staff often becomes a surrogate family to him or her. Tears are shed at times when patients recover and go home, just as tears are shed when they die.

Janet thinks that congregations and clergy have been slow to accept their responsibility to people with AIDS, if they acknowledge any responsibility at all. Her Methodist training taught her that the love of God is extended to everyone, saint and sinner alike. The churches and clergy that decide who should be loved, or that restrict their compassion only to "respectable" people are being "hypocritical," according to Janet. Further, she complains that the people of God not only have disregarded people with AIDS; they also have neglected an opportunity to minister to the health care personnel who care for AIDS patients out of a sense of professional and personal duty. The staff has needs, spiritual and emotional, that are ignored by clergy and congregations. Thus, members of the health care team rely on one another for support. They literally are "burned out people looking to other burned out people for support." She realizes that it may be difficult for religious people to minister to men and women of whose sexuality or conduct they disapprove. Nevertheless, she thinks that it may be even more difficult for young adults to cope with the losses associated with their disease and to come to peace before they die. Social workers cannot do everything for patients and all the people related to them. In Janet's view, "who is better equipped to help patients and the people who care for and about them come to terms with the ultimate questions of life and death than the clergy and people of faith."

PAM

Pam is a social worker. She is fifty years old, married, and the mother of two children in their twenties. Since 1982 Pam has been working with AIDS patients and their families, lovers, and friends. Pam always has had a liberal view of the world. She knew homosexual men and women. But none was a close friend. When she began to work with people with AIDS, she had to reassess her views regarding homosexuality. She says, "This took less than a day. I was clear about my sexuality, my values, and the values of social work—self-determination and a nonjudgmental attitude toward clients." After this reexamination, people with AIDS became and remain to her people who are sick. All other descriptions are irrelevant.

Pam has led what she describes as a "homogenous life." She was brought up "properly." Nevertheless, by inclination and with the encouragement of her husband, Pam is a "liberated woman." Her ten years of experience in social work have helped her to see goodness in everyone. She has shared with her children stories of how people with AIDS have been mistreated by society, families, and friends. Pam is convinced that their mistreatment does not result solely from their disease. It stems in part from who they are, i.e., homosexuals or intravenous drug abusers. Her children, in agreement with Pam and her husband, view the mistreatment of people with AIDS as a seemingly endless series of tragedies. They all have become more sensitive to the plight of minorities. They are outraged by the condemnations of people with AIDS and homosexual men. And they have been amazed at the homosexual population's ability to exist or maintain self-esteem in such a hostile environment.

Pam's work with AIDS patients takes more time than her work with other patients. Often AIDS patients have fewer support networks. And because they are young and not supposed to be dying, they have more issues and questions to work through. In addition to these personal issues, Pam is often involved in trying to mediate family rifts stemming from the patient's homosexuality. At times the patient's family deserts him or her. Abandonment by family raises additional issues for her to address with a patient. Social pronouncements that "they" deserve the disease complicate matters. The unavailability of social services like nursing home care, hospice care, and Meals on Wheels undercuts a patient's will to live. And finally, the absence of spiritual support may convey to patients that not only do people not care about them, but God doesn't care as well.

Pam is frustrated by AIDS. It is a full-time disease for those who have it. It takes everything they have (emotionally, financially, physically, spiritually) to take care of themselves. They "fail to thrive." All their systems slow down. And when they begin to become demented, the patients realize it. Their sense of desperation increases. They lose control of their lives and their bodies. They often are angry and frustrated. So is Pam. She sometimes questions if keeping them alive longer is a service if it means that they are going to die more horrible deaths.

Most of Pam's clients are gay men. The issues that she addresses with patients who have been infected by nonsexual routes are different. Hemophiliac patients often are married and have children. Their concerns are similar to the concerns of patients with terminal cancer. Transfusion patients have a form of anger related to their sense of misfortune or being unlucky. Drug abuse patients are the most difficult to serve. They seem to be unwilling or unable to take care of themselves. And their hostility makes it difficult at times to find out-of-hospital support people. Nevertheless, Pam sympathizes with the situations of all her patients. She has been impressed with the strength of human spirit displayed by people with AIDS. Despite overwhelming obstacles, they somehow have a drive to go on, to face and conquer adversity, and to cope as well as they can. Her young clients are not supposed to have the maturity to do all this. But on the whole, if they didn't have it when they became ill, they learn or develop it quickly.

Pam is realistic about the fate of her clients with AIDS—they all die sooner or later. She had to accept this before she could work with them constructively. In a sense, only after she accepted the inevitability of their deaths was she freed to help them live. Nevertheless, each death is a loss for her. She mourns them all.

The attitude and response of the federal government to AIDS angers Pam. She thinks that in relation to the magnitude of the present and potential suffering and death caused by AIDS, little money has been committed to the fight against it. She is pleased that money has been appropriated for research. She is upset, however, that no money has been allocated for patient care. Like other people reported in this book, Pam thinks that more money and other forms of support would have been forthcoming had AIDS first appeared in a population other than gay men. Had so-called innocents been affected first, the response of government, medicine, and the churches would not have been so slow, small and moralistic.

Pam thinks that the failure of a family to support a patient often stems from the inability to accept a son's or brother's homosexuality. Many parents have told her, "He's not my son anymore. He made his choice between his life-style and his family. We've made ours." Pam notes, however, that only fathers have been this rejecting. Some mothers and fathers don't desert their sons, but believe that their sons have brought their troubles on themselves. The parents apparently think that their sons intentionally put themselves at risk for AIDS by being gay and sexually active, a view that Pam rejects. Nevertheless, Pam is sensitive to the embarrassment, hurt, anger, and frustration that parents sometimes feel. They suffer alone—at times by choice. They refuse to share their burden with others. Some will go to great lengths to be certain that none of their friends discover the truth about their sons. Some ask that AIDS not appear on the death certificate. Others tell friends that their sons have cancer when they don't. Some parents have buried their sons' bodies away from their homes rather than risk an inadvertent discovery of the truth.

Pam becomes important to many of the patients. Her acceptance of them, obvious concern, and age results in her being seen by some patients as a surrogate mother. Pam remembers one case in particular. The patient was obnoxious. He refused to believe that Pam could help him work through his feelings. Pam and the patient were strong-willed. They hung on to each other. After six months of working on his feelings, needs, and inadequacies, the patient discovered his strengths of character. As his condition worsened, he decided against further life-support interventions. The patient said good-bye to his family and friends. He intended to die at home. By Thursday afternoon he was in such distress that he doubted he could die comfortably at home. He was admitted to the hospital. Pam went to see him in his room. He looked at Pam and said, "I'm dying." They talked. Pam went home. She expected the patient to die during the night. The next morning she was called to his room. She went in. He looked at her and said, "I'll die now." He closed his eyes and died immediately.

Pam's Protestant church was a big part of her life until seven years ago. She enjoyed working with the youth. But when she started her career as a social worker in a cancer hospital, her participation in the life of the congregation flagged. Pam felt that her fellow parishioners thought she was weird to enjoy working with cancer and death. She began to feel isolated. Her peers and her pastor seemed to do what they could to deny that life contained anything unpleasant. Suburban bliss was simply out of touch, in her mind, with the hard-core realities of finitude and vulnerability. Feeling out of place, Pam and her husband stopped attending worship.

Her anger at church people intensifies when homosexual people are condemned. Pam does not want to assume the position of God to decide who is and who is not acceptable. In her mind, if ability to love and depth of commitment to others are criteria, then, on the whole, gay couples and homosexual people compare favorably with straight couples or heterosexual people. Pam's God is loving and forgiving. Her work with AIDS patients has strengthened this perception of God. In her mind, Jesus is like God. Jesus didn't condemn an adulterous woman. Neither should Christians condemn people who they believe have committed a sexual sin. If sinlessness were a condition to be loved or to receive compassionate health care, then no one would pass. Pam would like to see the people of God be less judgmental and more compassionate in the AIDS crisis. People with AIDS need to be touched. They need to know that they count, that people care about them, not because they are gay or because they have AIDS, but because they are people who are sick. The ministry of the church should be comprehensive, spiritual and physical. AIDS, for Pam, is an opportunity for the church to mature, to broaden its belief about who is acceptable to God. The gap between what Christians say that they believe and what they do is wide, according to Pam. AIDS gives congregations a chance to narrow this gap. The congregations and the people with AIDS that they serve will both benefit from the experience.

MARK

Mark, a registered nurse, is co-owner of a firm that provides home health care. His involvement with people with AIDS has been brief. Nevertheless, in two years he has formulated some strong opinions about AIDS and the way people with AIDS are treated.

Mark began to care for AIDS patients because it seemed that other firms in his industry refused to do so. Care was denied because personnel feared infection, managers feared losing other business, and many patients were not insured and unable to pay for services. Mark and his partner made a commitment to serve this population. They saw a parallel between drug addicts and people with AIDS; both bear a social and moral stigma. As such, they are more easily ignored without an outcry of protest. Mark and his business partner disagreed with this line of thinking. They felt that someone needed to make a statement about the legitimacy of these people and respond to their needs for nurturing. They wanted to do what they could to transform people with AIDS from health care outcasts into the normal role of patient.

Adequately caring for AIDS patients requires maturer personnel, in Mark's mind. The normal care-givers and support systems of family, friends, hospitals, and physicians may not be there. The few people who are there, as a result of the absence of others, may have to assume a greater burden of care. In Mark's words, "It's a pathetic situation. I've never seen a group of people abandoned like this except drug addicts. Being alone makes it harder for some of the patients to work through their anger. They were never told that having sex with someone would kill you. They feel blind-sided. They often need help to sort through feelings of being cheated."

Mark has found his work with AIDS patients rewarding. Each patient enriches Mark's view of the world and humanity. Patients tend to want to talk, to tell him who they are and what makes them tick. The variety of experiences and the diversity of characters that he observes teach him about the strength of the human spirit.

Mark thinks that nearly all terminally ill patients reach a point where they really begin to live. They, perhaps for the first time, embody or personify abstractions like love, trust, equality, friendship. For most people, these are concepts for discussion. For terminal patients, the discovery of these attributes or qualities in themselves or others makes life meaningful even in the midst of dying.

Even though people with AIDS, like other patients with a fatal illness, seem able to affirm life as they anticipate death, they seem unique in their concern about what will happen after they die. The concerns that Mark identifies are not spiritual. AIDS patients seem inordinately concerned about their remains. They wonder, "Will anyone handle my body after I'm dead? Will I just lie here and rot? Will my wishes to be cremated be respected? Will my possessions be distributed as I want?" Some patients worry about the effect AIDS will have on their families. They hope their families will find the support they need. Some actually hope to develop Kaposi's sarcoma so their families can tell others that the diagnosis is cancer and, as a result, not be ostracized by others or endure a self-imposed isolation in their grief.

Mark, too, grieves the illness and death of his patients. He feels that he puts some of himself into each patient. Each patient, in turn, becomes part of him. When a patient dies he feels a double-edged loss, a loss of the patient and a loss of part of himself. Mark, like many of the people who care for people with AIDS, feels that he never has time to grieve properly. The deaths are too many and too often. "It would be nice," he says, "to find a group of people who would be willing to talk with me and others about the day-to-day stresses and griefs associated with caring for people with AIDS." He thinks that the social and religious condemnations of people with AIDS and the disvaluing of the people who try to help them make it unlikely that his need will be met by religious congregations. This doesn't necessarily bother him. He left his Christian congregation when he was sixteen years old. He didn't feel a need to participate in the church then and doesn't feel a need to participate now.

DOUG

Doug finished a residency in internal medicine in 1984 and began to specialize in AIDS in September 1985. Doug's professional interest, however, in gay sexuality began in 1978 when he accepted himself as a gay man. He helped to organize Gay and Lesbian People in Medicine, a support and social organization for homosexual people working in the health care professions. Further, Doug saw a need for more effective venereal services for gay men. He joined forces with other interested people to establish a clinic for gay men in Houston. Looking back, Doug thinks that these activities provided a good background for his involvement with the "ultimate sexually transmitted disease."

Doug saw his first patient with AIDS in July 1982. Little was understood about the disease then. He felt helpless. There were so many sophisticated tools available, but nothing seemed to help. What he saw was so awful that he "denied" AIDS would ever become the problem it has. As AIDS became more and more a problem for gay men, Doug felt "compelled" to focus his career on it. He believes that, as a physician who is gay, he is better able to understand the problems and the individuals most affected by the disease. Also, Doug feels an obligation to care for a population that few others will care for.

Doug thinks that caring for people with AIDS is different and more difficult than caring for other people with chronic or terminal diseases for the following reasons: (a) AIDS patients carry a stigma because of the disease or the at-risk population (gay or intravenous drug abuser) of which they are a member. Thus, people with AIDS are made to feel guilty for being ill, whereas most other patients are considered blameless. (b) Most people with AIDS are young. They tend to have little financial resources to soften the blow of lost income. Other patients in similar situations tend to be older, with more substantial assets. (c) AIDS patients are less likely when single to have someone at home to assist in their care. A patient who has a spouse and children has someone at home to help. (d) Much remains unknown about AIDS. The course of the disease and its complications are unpredictable. Most other chronic or fatal diseases are better understood. More knowledge about a disease enables physicians to help patients and others to understand what is happening. Where this is not possible, the disbelief, fear, and anger for everyone concerned are more acute. (e) It is more difficult to get support personnel to care for people with AIDS in and out of the hospital. This is less often the case for patients with other diagnoses.

These particularities of caring for people with AIDS can make the task more frustrating for the people who undertake it. The objective of care changes with AIDS, according to Doug. He feels that, in his words, "I can't get ahead of the game. All I can do is break even, not win. One thing after another happens. It never ends until the patient dies. And knowing that they are *all* going to die, despite everything I can do, increases the stress of my work. After all, most of them are around my age. People our age aren't supposed to be this sick or have such a high rate of death. Medical school didn't prepare me for this."

Despite the stress and grief that have become Doug's constant companions, he derives great satisfaction from his work. He tries to spend as much time as possible with each patient. They seem reassured if their condition is stable. He answers their questions as well as he can. Gaining information seems to relieve their anxiety. They are enabled to live more normally knowing what they can expect and what they can and cannot do. For example, Doug remembers the relief a young woman felt when she was told that using condoms was a way to be reasonably safe and be sexually active. Doug thinks that most of his patients "feel better" after they see him. This "feeling better" is important to the patients and gratifying to him.

Doug is currently encouraged by the federal, scientific, and medical responses to AIDS. It appears to him that some of the best scientists in the country are trying to solve the problem, but perhaps not solely for altruistic reasons. Nevertheless, the increase in federal funding is applauded, even though Doug resents the fact that it didn't come sooner. The present level of activity, in Doug's mind, should have begun before now. Governmental responses on the state and local levels have been "scandalous" across the nation. Politicians at every level, according to Doug, should interpret funding for research and care as a public health action, not an endorsement or condemnation of any life-style.

Doug also laments how some physicians have reacted to AIDS. As physicians, they should be able to set aside their personal biases and prejudices in order to respond to AIDS in the same way they would to any other disease. Disappointingly, this has not always been the case. Many physicians are providing high-quality,

165

compassionate care. But Doug has heard many stories from patients about being turned away. Also scandalous to Doug is the use by some physicians of their medical license to authorize and justify a personal and political agenda to deny homosexual people their rights.

Doug's family knows about his work. They also know that he is gay and lives with his lover. At first his father was concerned about the risks to Doug from his work. After these questions were answered he supported Doug's commitment. His friends, gay and straight, also support him and his work. They are amazed by some of the stories he tells of how badly some patients are treated by their families or friends and by the devastation of the disease. They ask, "How can you stand to work with that all day long?" Doug's answer is straightforward: "It's what I must do." The tragedies associated with AIDS cause him to want to be part of the fight to overcome it. Again, in his words, "AIDS itself is a tragedy. But when people are rejected by their families and endure the indignities of proposals for quarantine, extermination, and God knows what next, the disease and the unkind human response to the people who suffer it become an abomination."

The understanding and support of his family has been important to Doug as he affirmed his sexuality and shaped his career. He wishes that all, rather than some, of his gay patients with AIDS received the same sort of familial affirmation. Also, he wishes that employers and co-workers of people with AIDS would react sympathetically, rather than tell the sick, but able to work, person to go home. The isolation associated with AIDS is not limited to patients. The same fears that prompt people to reject patients are known to family members of patients. As a result, they often do all they can to "cover up" the family secret. Keeping the truth unknown can become a major task if a son or daughter returns home.

Not only does the parents' physical burden increase, but also old conflicts between parent and child can be resurrected as the parent-infant role is reestablished to the displeasure of everyone.

Doug's Southern Baptist background largely is irrelevant to him now. Nevertheless, he recognizes that religious faith is important to many people, including some of his patients and their families. Doug thinks that congregations have an obligation to care for and provide supports for these patients and families. Congregations can become educated about AIDS and the potential needs of all people touched by AIDS as a first step in responding to AIDS. Then congregations should, in Doug's words, "get their hands dirty." They should be with families and patients, doing with them whatever is indicated in order to confirm the congregation's care and support of them. These services or ministries, when done by the members of the congregation, are much more meaningful to the people affected most directly by AIDS than if they were provided by strangers paid by the congregation. Doug believes, drawing on his training as a child, that if one accepts the biblical witness concerning Jesus' teaching and conduct, the sort of ministry he envisages is an obligation, not an option.

ROGER

Roger's twenty-five-year career as a physician has been one of changing interests and developing new competencies. His intellectual and humanitarian involvements have taken him to Great Britain, Africa, Canada, and the United States. His original training as a surgeon has evolved into specialties in internal medicine, immunology, and virology. Roger is divorced. His four children live with their mother in Canada. His interests and activities are many, including the arts, gourmet cooking, gardening, and volunteer activities such as feeding homeless men and women. Roger also enjoys reading. Books on theology, philosophy, and ethics are in his library. Although he does not characterize himself as expert in these disciplines, a knowledge of them is considered essential to his understanding of life, disease, death, and his role as a physician.

Roger's personal stake in AIDS began in 1981, when an employee developed a yeast infection in his mouth. At that time AIDS was first being described. Roger thought that immunosuppression was a less important problem to solve than the Kaposi's sarcoma that he was seeing. Then Roger began to see people with opportunistic infections. Next he saw people with ARC, and others who were symptom-free but had evidence of being immunocompromised. The evidence mounted that AIDS was an infectious disease theoretically treatable by antiviral drugs.

As Roger began to see more and more people with AIDS, his early hope that the problem would be solved within a short time began to fade. Since 1982, when Roger restricted his work to AIDS, he and his two colleagues have seen hundreds of people with AIDS, most of them young gay men. Because of his involvement with pediatric oncology, he was not unfamiliar with young people dying. But with AIDS, the patients deteriorated quickly. Young adults who were educated, delightful, artistic, and cultured were being struck down. It all seemed so senseless and wasteful. Roger's anger and frustration grew as he observed the way AIDS affects people and with his inability to do much about it therapeutically, except to be a sustaining presence.

No disease that he knows is quite as devastating as is AIDS to the people who suffer it. Indeed, other diseases kill. But AIDS, in Roger's mind, is unique because of the scope and severity of its nonphysical consequences. First, people with AIDS dominantly are members of an ostracized group, i.e., gay men. They tend not to be respected and are even maligned. Their self-image and self-esteem have been battered by an unaccepting society, and perhaps by an unaccepting family. When they contract a disease that evokes a fearful, hostile, recriminating response, their feelings about themselves are further lowered. The guilt and regret that people with AIDS often feel, at least at diagnosis and soon after, are greater, in Roger's opinion, than that felt by people whose fatal illness is related to their behavior (e.g., smoking and lung cancer). Second, people with AIDS tend to fear more the consequences of their diagnosis unrelated to their physical decline than do patients with other fatal diseases. They fear, for example, the immediate loss of employment, friends, family, insurance, and housing. And third, people may isolate, reject, neglect, and abuse people with AIDS with legal and moral impunity.

These factors join with others to make efforts medically to treat people with AIDS a frustrating endeavor for Roger and his patients. It is frustrating to observe psychiatric and neurological complications, including blindness, and be able to do little or nothing about them. It is frustrating when patients who have compromised immune systems fail to respond to drugs as expected. It is frustrating not to be able to obtain appropriate, unapproved drugs in a timely fashion. It is frustrating to deal with other physicians who seem indifferent to the plight of people with AIDS. It is frustrating not to have other physicians respect one's work. It is frustrating not to make a major discovery that advances care. It is frustrating to be treated badly at times by patients who are angry and frustrated themselves. Finally, it is frustrating to work in a political climate that withholds resources necessary to meet patients' needs.

Despite these frustrations, Roger perseveres with his work. It is intellectually satisfying to be working on a fascinating medical problem. The uncertainty can also bring rewards, like finding an unknown parasite in a patient's stool. So sometimes Roger feels like an explorer. But most satisfying to Roger is the relationship he has with some of the patients. Many become good friends. Their deaths are especially difficult to accept. But there have been hundreds of others whom Roger has come to respect and admire. In the midst of their illness they have an interest in him as a person. They talk about other subjects, in addition to their medical complaints, when they visit. Roger looks forward to their coming. When they leave the office something of them remains with him. When they die a part of Roger dies. Roger finds it impossible not to reciprocate with a similar personal interest and investment of himself in them.

Because of Roger's concern for people with AIDS and his interest in competent, compassionate medical care, he is intolerant of physicians who refuse to treat or who mistreat these patients rather than refer in order to collect a fee. Similarly, he is intolerant of drug companies that misrepresent the efficacy of their drugs, exploiting the desperation of patients in order to increase profits. Finally, Roger is intolerant of passive aggressive behavior by consulting physicians who refuse to do indicated procedures at an inconvenient time, e.g., Friday afternoon, when they would otherwise if the patient did not have AIDS.

Roger yearns for the discovery of an antiviral agent, immune restorative agent, or some combination of the two that will end the devastation and death. In the interim, prevention of the disease by avoiding the known risk factors is indicated. However, according to Roger, people continue to smoke cigarettes and drive while drunk despite the known risks. Thus, education and behavior modification probably won't eliminate all future cases. A vaccine would be ideal. But as of now, no vaccine is in sight. Moreover, a vaccine won't help the thousands of people who now have AIDS, the hundreds of thousands who have ARC, or the millions of people who have been infected with the AIDS virus and whose futures are unknown

While biomedical scientists and physicians search for a cure and try to help patients have as long and qualitative a life as possible, Roger thinks that the church has a unique and important contribution to make to people with AIDS. The church has the unique ability to provide a form of nonphysical comfort and consolation to people who must deal with, what he designates, "the imponderables of life." Physicians, psychiatrists, nurses, and social workers do not have the depth of knowledge that well-read clergy do to respond adequately or authoritatively to questions like "Why is this happening? What does it mean?" People with AIDS have these questions. The church and its clergy, in Roger's mind, should be there to talk with patients about them.

But patients are not the only people involved with AIDS who have these questions. He also does. Other professional personnel do. Families of patients do. Lovers and friends of patients do. Roger thinks that for the church to abdicate its mission in this crisis is to do itself and everyone concerned a disservice. Even though Roger left the Episcopal Church fifteen years ago because he no longer felt it met any of his needs, he retains an interest to explore with reasoned and reasonable clergy and lay people the apparent contradiction between conceiving God as a compassionate being and the

171

phenomenon of human suffering. He believes that a compassionate God wills the relief of suffering. As a physician combating suffering, Roger feels that he is aligned with God. Nevertheless, his sense of unity of purpose with God does not cause him to feel drawn to churches and people in them who seem willing to ignore, even compound, the suffering of people with AIDS and those related to them.

STEVE

Steve's medical specialties are oncology and internal medicine. Steve started practice at a Health Maintenance Organization (HMO) in 1981, the same year that young gay men began to appear with opportunistic infections and Kaposi's sarcoma. As a cancer specialist, Steve was involved in the care of the first few patients with Kaposi's sarcoma at his HMO. He was impressed by how similar these patients were to patients with acute leukemia. Figuratively speaking, one minute they would be completely well, and the next minute they would be short of breath, have an elevated temperature, and require immediate hospitalization. And despite doing everything possible, they died. Steve felt the same way about acute leukemia patients and AIDS patients—helpless. This feeling exists even now, five year later.

AIDS, as a disease, interested Steve as a scientist and a clinician. Trying to understand AIDS and cancer is an intriguing intellectual exercise. But on the affective, emotional level, Steve feels that caring for people with AIDS can be a genuine privilege. He has had to defend his aggressive treatment of AIDS patients against the objections of his colleagues at the HMO. Some of them say, "Why bother? They're dead already. Save the clinic some money. They're a drain on the clinic. Only do what you must to keep them comfortable." Steve feels that he cannot professionally or personally comply with his colleagues' requests to minimize care and, as a result, maximize profits.

Like the AIDS population in general, the majority of Steve's patients with AIDS are gay men ("one of the boys," as they are called by Steve's colleagues). Their homosexuality is not an issue to Steve, who has several close friends who are gay. The person who was best man at his wedding, a fellow oncologist, is gay. Alternate life-styles have never offended him or caused him to feel less of a duty to care medically for people who live them. He has been offended, however, by the discrimination expressed toward homosexual people. The tragedies associated with AIDS have strengthened his commitment to fight against oppressive and discriminating practices against homosexual people. The extent of Steve's acceptance and support of homosexual people is indicated by his attendance at gay union services and the friendship that Steve and his wife have with some of the lovers and families of his AIDS patients.

Some of Steve's friends have expressed surprise that he allows a dead AIDS patient's lover to give gifts to his infant daughter, play with her, and kiss her on the cheek. But Steve acts in a manner consistent with his scientific knowledge of the AIDS virus. He is convinced that this sort of conduct is no risk to his daughter. Further, he believes that he is at no great risk when he cares for his patients as long as he takes adequate precautions when indicated. Steve's AIDS patients seem to understand that he cares for them, is open to them, and accepts them. His concern for them as persons causes him to establish bonds with them. The bond is strongest with patients that he has known for the longest time. So when they suffer or die, Steve grieves. He finds it impossible and does not desire to guard against this inevitability.

Steve admires the strength of character and resolve of many of his patients. One patient has had AIDS for two years. His course has been complex. He has had *Pneumocystis carinii* pneumonia four times. He has chronic viral and protozoan infections in his bowel that cause unrelenting diarrhea. He also has a chronic herpes infection. For the past eighteen months this patient has been nourished by fluids infused into a subclavian vein. The patient and his lover, who has ARC, are devoted to each other. In Steve's mind, their love for each other sustains them. The patient with AIDS goes to work every day. Not to go to work, in his mind, is equivalent to giving up, to dying.

Another patient displayed the same perseverance. He was a strong man with a sensitive soul and artistic hands. He made stained-glass windows for his living. And despite his overwhelming physical problems, he was always doing small things for other people. Steve became friends with this patient and his lover. When the lovers visited Steve at home, they would bring a gift to his daughter. On one occasion they drove fifty miles to buy a Cabbage Patch doll for Steve's daughter. This young man fought to live until the last week of his life, when he could fight no longer. He wanted to and did die at home with his lover by his side. The man's lover called Steve to tell him as he cried, "Your patient has died." Steve responded, "Kiss him good-bye for me." Had he been there, Steve says, that is what he would have done. After he placed the receiver in its carriage, Steve sat down to cry.

Steve hopes that the day will soon come when he can discharge patients who are cured rather than dead. He notes that much progress has been made in understanding the underlying immune disorder of AIDS and treating the disorders caused by it. Steve thinks that a major breakthrough will occur within five years. When it comes it will have far-reaching implications for other medical problems. The whole field of cancer treatment will change. Learning how to turn the immune system on and off or bolster it will open new avenues to treat a range of problems from infection to rejection of organ implants. Steve thinks that if people understood the benefits to everyone that may emerge from research involving people with AIDS and care for them, perhaps there would be a more tolerant, understanding, and compassionate response now. Further, perhaps more funds would be available for research and treatment. In short, according to Steve, it's in everyone's interest that this occur.

While a cure for AIDS is being sought, Steve will continue to fight for the lives, rights, and dignity of his patients. He is alarmed by calls for mass screenings of people to detect antibody to the AIDS virus. As far as he is concerned, these are thinly veiled efforts to discriminate against gay men. He has one patient whose employer discovered that the patient has been infected by the AIDS virus. Even though the patient is clinically healthy, he has not been allowed to return to work. This patient is lucky. He continues to receive full pay. Other people are not so lucky. They lose their jobs, insurance, and future. These forms of overt and covert discrimination bias Steve to people with AIDS and the populations at risk for AIDS, principally gay men.

Steve finds himself spending more and more time with his patients with AIDS. He knows that at present the war is lost. But he also knows that battles can be won. He celebrates these short-term victories but remains committed to winning the war. He wants to win for the people now living with AIDS, not only for the general population that the Reagan Administration seems primarily concerned to protect. Steve frankly is cynical about the sincerity of the Reagan Administration's putative concern for the predominantly gay men who now suffer with this disease.

Steve's identification with oppressed and persecuted people is due partly to his religious commitments. He was brought up in a Protestant congregation but dropped out during college. When Steve's father died eight years ago he felt a need to explore religion again. He studied Eastern religions, Protestant and Catholic Christianity, and Judaism. Steve was drawn to Conservative Judaism. He became a converted Jew at thirty-four years of age. His new religion has helped him to feel a solidarity with and have compassion for any persecuted population. Because he believes that God sides with people who are treated unjustly, he should too. Every congregation, Jewish or Christian, sooner or later will have to face AIDS, the isolation it evokes, and the horrors it produces. Steve thinks that congregations are in a unique position to organize and alleviate some of the unnecessary pain and suffering. To quote Steve after a moment of reflection, "Do you think they will?"

Pastoral Perspectives and Recommendations

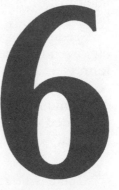

The suffering that AIDS has wrought is incalculable. The pain, worry, exhaustion, dependency, loss, grief, and death portrayed in the preceding pages is representative of the human devastation associated with this fear-evoking disease. In situations where indifference, insensitivity, and isolation are too common, it is perhaps remarkable that there have been instances where the affected people have found comfort and peace in the midst of tragedy. If the stories in this book are indicative of the general situation, it appears that whatever victories have been won in the midst of defeat have been realized largely apart from the participation of the people of God. The near-total failure of the church to fulfill its theologically and biblically mandated role in these crises of illness and death raises questions about the integrity of contemporary American Christendom. Indeed, AIDS, or any fatal disease, arouses fear. But the fear evoked by other diseases, even fatal ones, has not prevented the church from implementing compassionate and supportive ministries to the people who suffer them and to their loved ones. In this sense, AIDS has engendered a unique inaction by the church, an inaction that does nothing to unite people who are estranged

177

(the church and the at-risk populations) and insulates itself from the anguish of the reconciled (church members).

A redemptive response to AIDS would appear possible, even required, if the teaching in the First Epistle of John were taken seriously. The several fears that partly account for the societal and ecclesiastical response to AIDS might be overcome by courage and compassion grounded in divine love if the counsel of First John were heeded.

> There is no room for fear in love; perfect love banishes fear. For fear brings with it the pains of judgement, and anyone who is afraid has not attained to love in its perfection. We love because he loved us first. But if a man says, "I love God," while hating his brother, he is a liar. If he does not love the brother whom he has seen, it cannot be that he loves God whom he has not seen. And indeed this command comes to us from Christ himself: that he who loves God must also love his brother. (1 John 4:18–21, NEB)

The question that AIDS presents to the church is basically one of its identity. In short, is the church a redemptive, loving servant people serving a servant Lord?[1] The true question for the church has nothing to do with the morality of certain conduct or the status before God of certain people associated with AIDS (cf. Galatians 6:10). These issues are secondary, at best, to the primary issue of the integrity and credibility of the people who bear Christ's name. For people who claim Jesus as Lord to neglect the opportunities for ministry generated by AIDS constitutes a failure in discipleship. Individual Christians and the Body of Christ have no option. The "outcast," the person with AIDS and people related to him or her, must be loved with the same unmeasured love that Jesus embodied. For those who claim the name of Christ, this is the only acceptable attitude, and it ought to produce appropriate reconciling and compassionate ministries.

As the stories presented here indicate, people with AIDS come from all walks of life. They are sons, daughters, fathers, mothers, brothers, and sisters who are now suffering and dying because of one or more inadvertent infections with a virus that progressively destroys the body's capacity to defend itself. They are people with feelings, needs, hopes, and dreams. They are related to people by birth or by choice who care about them. Patients are not the only people who suffer and grieve the multiple losses directly or indirectly caused by AIDS. Natural and chosen families, friends (whether they flee or abide), and health care personnel suffer in their own ways. The suffering and grief associated with any fatal illness are compounded in the case of AIDS because of the stigmas attached to the disease and the primary at-risk populations. As a result, there have been few expressions of sympathy or compassion by people who claim moral and political leadership in the United States. Instead, people with AIDS are said to deserve their diseases. Public support is undermined and the work of people who provide care is disparaged as a consequence. The situation is unconscionable in secular life and lamentable in the life of the church.

As the number of people with AIDS grows, it will become increasingly unlikely that individual congregations throughout the nation will remain untouched. As of March 1986 there were approximately 9,000 persons alive with AIDS. Perhaps 180,000 additional persons are diagnosed with ARC. And it is conservatively estimated that about 2 million persons have been infected with the AIDS virus. Despite efforts to control the transmission of the virus, epidemiologists project that the number of people with AIDS and related conditions will continue to increase rapidly. Add to these present and projected figures the number of people who are likely to be affected because of their relationship to an infected individual and the magnitude of potential suffering caused by AIDS increases dramatically. In short, AIDS is not now, nor will it be, only an urban problem. Gay men, intravenous drug abuse, and heterosexual prostitution may be concentrated in cities, but they are not exclusively urban phenomena. Further, the parents, siblings, children, grandparents, aunts, uncles, cousins, and friends of people with AIDS or ARC can be and are found all across the country. It seems reasonable to conclude, therefore, that almost no congregation will totally escape the impact of AIDS. The needs of people for pastoral care and other supportive ministries surely will increase. Similarly, opportunities for a variety of ministries to patients, loved ones, and health care personnel will increase. The implied and explicit pleas for the church to be a more active participant in ameliorating the suffering caused by AIDS predictably will grow in number and intensity as more and more people are directly or indirectly affected. The church cannot legitimately ignore or withdraw from the challenges and opportunities for ministry presented by AIDS. It must not only be present to and serve people who suffer, but it must also take up its prophetic mantle to remind itself and society of obligations under God to the "outcast" and the "oppressed," the "powerless" and the "poor."[2]

PERSPECTIVES ON PEOPLE WITH AIDS OR ARC

The stories presented in chapter 3 illustrate why it is appropriate to characterize people with AIDS or ARC as contemporary instances of the "dispossessed" and the "poor" who were the subjects of benevolent prophetic concern in Israel (Exodus 22:21–22; Jeremiah 34:8–14) and in the teaching and ministry of Jesus (Matthew 25:31–46). This generalization appears true for the AIDS and ARC populations as a whole, but there are notable exceptions in each. Not all who are stricken by the AIDS virus are abandoned and despised by people who are meaningful to them. Nevertheless, the risk of rejection and isolation, even quarantine, is ever present. As control of their bodies and lives slips away, their dependency on others increases. Their fears that their care-providers will wear out before they finally die can be intense. Thus, they attempt to remain independent for as long as possible. This may mean that their diagnosis and periods of illness are kept secret until it is impossible to do so.

Another reason for maintaining secrecy is a desire to protect others from truths that may be difficult or impossible to bear. Family members, particularly parents of gay people with AIDS or ARC, may be kept in the dark. Perceptions by siblings that parents cannot handle certain disclosures regarding a son's sexuality or illness often result in a conspiracy to deny them this information. These efforts tend to be undertaken out of a concern to protect people from hurt. Similarly, people with AIDS or ARC may refuse new relationships in order to minimize their own losses and protect people from the grief caused by the patient's death. These protective actions are understandable, but they may result in a self-imposed isolation that limits the quality and quantity of care that patients receive. When this is the case, people who wish to minister to people with AIDS or ARC may need to demonstrate not only their desire, but also their commitment to be present to and with them until the end.

Disappointment and grief are common emotions

among people with AIDS or ARC. Gay men, in particular, have had to wrestle with discoveries about who they are as sexual beings in an unaccepting, condemning cultural and ecclesiastical environment. The resiliency with which they negotiated this discovery and subsequent personal declaration may have been a helpful preparation for negotiating the additional discovery of having ARC or AIDS. In addition, their capacity to withstand cultural condemnation may have helped to equip them to withstand the indifferent and hostile reactions to the disease that they embody. Despite these assaults on self-esteem, it seems remarkable that within the gay AIDS and ARC populations almost no one regrets being homosexual. These gay men maintain, almost without exception, a pride about themselves. Their self-acceptance may insulate them from the losses that so often accompany AIDS, but it does not fully protect them from the hurt that follows rejection or failing loyalties.

Their losses are many, severe, and rapid. Nevertheless, in a situation where almost everything is being taken away, people with AIDS develop and express a concern for others who also, or may not, have AIDS or ARC. This may be a component of their desire to "take care of business" or "put things right" before they die. Or, more accurately, in our opinion, it results from a need, and perhaps newly found ability, to put life in perspective. AIDS, or any fatal disease, reminds persons who have it that time, like life, is a precious possession. If they are to make sense of life, death, morality, or God, they must do it promptly. Almost without exception in our experience, the people with AIDS or ARC have pursued this task without the benefit of clergy, Christian laity, or philosophers. Either they selectively have drawn on religious training as children to come to peace with themselves, life, and God, or they have set aside childhood religious memories and found consolation elsewhere. In either case, the effort to derive meaning from experience—their experience—is nearly universal. It seems that in this pilgrimage they experience a form of liberation uncommon among people not facing their own deaths. In short, by accepting death as their fate, they are freed to live (cf. Mark 8:34–35). And in the process, some discover or develop strengths of character and insights into the nature of the human condition that were previously unknown to them.

It may be that most people who contemplate ultimate questions as they await their foreseen or imminent deaths become philosophers or theologians. The people with AIDS or ARC reported here (and others known to the authors) almost without exception felt some need for God. Their conceptions of God vary, as do their understandings of divine moral judgment. Some ideas, beliefs, and practices seem bizarre, others appear more orthodox. The variety of religious thought and expression seems less significant than the implicit or explicit felt need to relate to God (however deity is conceived and perceived by the dying person). It may be that people with AIDS or ARC, as a group, do not feel a need to be related to institutionalized churches that closed their doors to them when they were well, because of their sexuality.

Press reports of television preachers and other religious leaders claiming that AIDS is God's punishment on homosexuality and America say to homosexual and AIDS populations that the welcome sign on the church door does not apply to them. This view of God's relation to AIDS is nearly uniformly rejected by people directly or indirectly affected by this disease. In this sense they evidence a greater degree of theological profoundness and sophistication than the "Christian celebrities" who see AIDS as divine retribution on a sinful people. People with AIDS, therefore, take refuge directly in God, rather than in the institutions and with the people who claim to represent God.

When AIDS is conceived as God's punishment, people may feel justified to turn away and let the "dead bury the dead." This sort of thinking is at odds with Jesus' command for his disciples to heal the sick (Mark 6:7–13). At this time, total physical healing or cure is beyond reach. But there are other forms of healing in which Christians can participate, including healings of the spirit and of broken relationships.[3] This may require Christians to see and feel the way people do who bear the stigma of the AIDS virus (cf. Luke 10:33). After all, this is the meaning of compassion, to feel *with* another person. If this sort of identification should occur, perhaps some "careless" comments and actions that deepen the hurt that people with AIDS or ARC feel could be foregone. Being sensitive to how one's statements or conduct may be interpreted by another person, especially a person who is dying *and* stigmatized, is a basic component of caring for him or her. From the position and perspective of one who is losing or has lost control of his or her life (i.e., the "poor"), the special concern that God's servants are to have for the ostracized and alienated people (cf. Psalms 10:14–18; 113:7) may take on a new relevance and move God's people to undertake redemptive ministries to people caught in the AIDS crisis.

People with AIDS tend not to blame God for the appearance of the AIDS virus and its attack on their bodies. Similarly, people who contract AIDS by blood transfusion or the administration of blood products tend to blame neither God nor gay men. Why is it that some Christians and some segments of the public are willing to attribute AIDS to God and link it to God's alleged condemnation of homosexuality?[4] Although the answer to this question surely is complex and beyond the scope of this discussion, it seems reasonable to suggest that it is related to the fears discussed in the first chapter and, more specifically, the fears of sexuality and homosexuality.

The mistakenly perceived necessary link between AIDS and male homosexuality appears to be used by some people to legitimate societal prejudice and discrimination against gay men. In this sort of oppressive and unjust environment, Christians, according to the apostle Paul, are to be God's agents of justice, their bodies being "instruments of righteousness" (cf. Romans 6:12–14). A ministry that "sets right," comforts, and reconciles brokenness is required in response to AIDS. The means by which a person contracted the AIDS virus or his or her life-style does not lessen the obligation of the church to care for him or her. To the contrary, the fact that a person with AIDS or ARC is a homosexual or bisexual male, drug abuser, or prostitute may clarify and underscore the church's duty to befriend and defend him or her. Their status in society and their physical condition may mean that there is almost no one to care for them other than God and God's people. Because this tends to be the case, the church, if it is to be the church, must not abandon people with AIDS or ARC or be a party to society's neglect of them.

PERSPECTIVES ON FAMILIES AND LOVERS

As the stories of families and lovers reveal, the person with AIDS or ARC is not the only one who suffers. Everyone involved may feel trapped, impotent, and unable to alter the inevitable course of events. Like the patient, families often feel insecure and without supports. They tend to suffer and grieve alone because they fear that the stigma attached to the disease or to their loved one's life-style will be extended to them. They rightly or wrongly often bear their burden alone, not trusting church peers, neighbors, or relatives to understand their situation or act compassionately toward them. No other disease evokes this sort of isolation. As a result, families find comfort with strangers, either people who are sharing the same experience or caring professionals.

Families experience many forms of grief as a result of AIDS. Parents, for example, may lose their image of a son, their dream for grandchildren, or the security of a child's care during old age. And not least of all, they probably will lose their son or daughter. Parents and siblings also may lose friends if the situation of their loved one becomes known. They may lose social contacts and outlets if they participate in the care of a child or sibling whose dependency grows as the disease and its complications worsen.

The families who feel the most fear of disclosure and most isolated tend to be the ones whose loved one has AIDS and is part of a derogated group. The fear of loss or embarrassment may cause families to turn away from their son or daughter with AIDS. Religious judgments that AIDS is God's punishment or that homosexual conduct is sinful may be another reason to abandon one's kin. Fear can be a powerful emotion. It can cause people to say or do things that they would never imagine saying or doing. Similarly, love can be a powerful emotion. Love can cause people to overcome fear and certain religious convictions in order to abide with a loved one who has AIDS or with a loved one who has AIDS and carries an additional stigma as well, e.g., gay or bisexual male, drug abuser, prostitute.

Even if families do not reject or abandon their kin,

their experience with AIDS often remains private, and they fail to receive the care and support of people who in other circumstances would share their grief. This desire to protect themselves, or their loved one, from additional rebuke is not blameworthy. It illustrates the degree to which AIDS and its perceived correlates (e.g., male homosexuality) are negatively judged in contemporary life. These negative evaluations seem mistaken. AIDS is a disease, not in itself a moral issue. Homosexual is what some people discover themselves to be; again, not in itself a moral issue. Yet it appears that homosexuality is regarded as such a disgrace by some parents that spouses won't talk to each other about their suspicions regarding a child. Perhaps the concern here is to protect each other. If so, the silence is not blameworthy, only regrettable.

Lovers of gay men with AIDS or ARC also suffer. A lover in a homosexual union has a role equivalent to a spouse in a heterosexual marriage. The love between homosexual partners is comparable to the love between heterosexual partners. Thus, the feelings and emotions are comparable when one is ill or dying. The fear, worry, sadness, and grief are the same. Some factors, however, may compound the grief that normally would be expected in this situation. For example, homosexual relationships are not recognized in law. There may be conflicts between a lover and the patient's family, who, unless the patient has arranged otherwise, has legal authority to make decisions concerning the patient's care if he or she becomes unable to make decisions. Being deprived of this sort of responsibility at the end of a long struggle together can cause the surviving gay man to feel as if he has not fulfilled the duties associated with his role. In addition, he may not be the one to make arrangements regarding the disposition of the corpse. He may be denied participation in funeral or memorial services. Finally, wills and insurance policies may be contested by a family who refuses to recognize the relationship.

Another factor that can complicate matters is the level of care that people with AIDS or ARC may require for an extended time. Friends, for a variety of reasons, may disappear. Often the lover of a person with AIDS is forced to perform a balancing act. He may work to meet his own and the couple's combined living expenses. The full burden of household chores may fall to the healthy partner. In addition, he may be required to feed, bathe, medicate, and, perhaps, frequently diaper his lover. The cycle of work at his job and at home may be repeated day after day for weeks or months. The fatigue that often results from this schedule can lead to an unintentional neglect of the sick lover. The routine can lessen the care-giving lover's resistance to disease, thus heightening worry about his own health and continued ability to care for his lover. These personal health-related worries are typically added to concerns about previous infection by the AIDS virus during sexual activities.

Finally, a lover's situation may be worsened because of the need to keep his sexuality and relationship secret from people who, if he were in a heterosexual relationship and the disease was other than AIDS, would typically provide respite and other forms of support. Employer and co-workers, family, and friends may never be told what is happening. As a result, the isolation imposed by AIDS may become more concentrated. Pastoral care and congregational support may not be requested because of a desire to avoid another possible rejection or condemnation. In short, pastoral ministries by clergy or laity that could ameliorate the suffering of everyone involved often are missing in AIDS.

There are notable exceptions to these scenarios of

isolation and compounded grief. Some families and lovers tell all. Some families and lovers have mutual concern and respect for each other. Some pastors and congregants provide appropriate pastoral care and other support ministries. In some situations everyone involved respects and is sensitive to the needs and concerns of others. When this is the case, everyone seems to cope better with a seemingly endless series of losses. Most of all, the sick or dying person tends to receive the supportive care of lover and family, all of which may be essential to a peaceful death.

PERSPECTIVES ON PROFESSIONAL CARE-PROVIDERS

The professional personnel who provide medical, nursing, and psychosocial care to people with AIDS or ARC also suffer. Their involvements with patients can be intense. Care-providers frequently bond with patients. Somehow they manage to sort through their feelings about sexuality, disease, life-styles, and death as they converge in AIDS and remain loyal to patients. Care-providers who are not comfortable with people with AIDS or ARC tend to withdraw from their care. But the personnel who persevere somehow move beyond stereotypes and prejudices to view each patient as worthy of competent and respectful professional assistance. In the midst of perpetual illness and death, they manifest a deep and genuine compassion for hurting humanity. The investment of patient and care-provider in each other establishes a relationship in which professional objectivity may fail and vulnerabilities are laid bare. As a result of frequent meetings, pleasant and likeable patients can become friends. Their setbacks, losses, and deaths grieve the people who provide professional care. Even demanding, abusive, and generally unlikeable patients seem to gain the professional staff's sympathy, if not their respect and affection.

AIDS is an enigma to professional care-providers. The disease progresses in unpredictable ways. It dominantly affects people at an age when they are not supposed to die. Patients may experience several life-threatening illnesses at once, one or more of which may not respond to conventional therapies or not be therapeutically approachable. As a result, care-providers tend to be frustrated by not being able to cure or, at times, palliate. The quantity and intensity of services required by patients can be tiring. And stresses can mount as the death toll rises. In short, AIDS is unique in its ability to destroy patients and wear down people who work to defeat it.

Professional personnel who care for people with AIDS or ARC can have their energy drained, emotional balance upset, and religious beliefs challenged as a result of their work. The depleting character of their service to this population establishes in them a particular need for pastoral care and congregational support. Not only do their ministries ultimately fail, but their efforts may also be demeaned by peers and public who disvalue the populations primarily affected by the disease. They are reminded almost daily of their professional and personal limitations. They know better than anyone that they alone cannot meet the full range of needs that patients have. Realizing that a cure is not now available and that prolonging a patient's life may not, in actuality, be providing him or her with a qualitative existence, care-providers understand the value of comfort and consolation for patients, loved ones, and themselves. It may be, given the current state of affairs, that one of the most valuable contributions that everyone can make in the AIDS crisis is to be a "sustaining presence"[5] to the affected people. Each person in his or her role as lover, friend, parent, sibling, nurse, social worker, or physician can abide with the person with AIDS or ARC and with one another, demonstrating by one's presence and ministries that the patient is valued and valuable even though sick, dependent, or dying, and that all concerned are worthy of respect and compassionate support.

Few of the clinicians portrayed in this volume are actively involved in religious communities. Nevertheless, they all evidence a humanitarianism, compassion, and benevolence that one would like to think is characteristic of all people of faith. It may be that their disaffection from the church is partly responsible for their ability to reach out to the AIDS population. Their independence from culturally and ecclesiastically mediated prejudices and condemnations may have freed them to see the pain, fear, debilitation, suffering, and grief as embodied in persons rather than faceless stereotypes or depersonalized statistics. As a result of their involvement with patients, they have learned firsthand that the suffering caused by AIDS and ARC goes far beyond the number of actual cases. In light of the extent of suffering and the people of God's claim to be a loving community, they ask, where is the church and its people in this crisis? This is an obvious, yet profound, question that the church and its people answer either by active, compassionate ministries or by oversight or neglect. The unique ministries that the church can provide in this sort of crisis mostly would be welcomed by the people presently "in the trenches." Patients, loved ones, and care-providers want and need the consolation, comfort, and peace that the gospel and the people whose lives are shaped by it can bring to the situation.

RECOMMENDATIONS FOR PASTORAL AND CONGREGATIONAL MINISTRIES

AIDS confronts the church with new pastoral challenges. The invariably fatal outcome, the societal rejection of AIDS patients, and the social isolation many affected people experience combine to create a new situation for the church's ministry. All the consequences of this situation cannot be explicated here, but some observations can be made. First, the degree of isolation is directly related to the attempts by patients to preserve their diminishing privacy and self-respect. Because people with AIDS have come to expect social ostracism in their daily lives, they fear the additional antagonism and rejection they would face if their situation became known. The isolation of parents and siblings can be equally painful. They are reluctant to discuss their plight with pastors or members of their congregations, perhaps to protect their loved one or themselves from rejection. The lack of trust in clergy or lay people to feel and express compassion and acceptance is often a hallmark of comments by family members. In their loneliness, parents choose to bear this pain privately. Similarly, lovers and care-givers indicate that the general response of people to the at-risk populations conditions them to expect rejection by congregations or representatives of religious communities. It is this characteristic of the AIDS epidemic that is unique from any previous pastoral care opportunity, and as such makes the situation a challenge. The situation calls for a pastoral response that reconciles.

Second, the pastoral care movement has been chided for providing an appropriate supportive ministry to people in emotional crisis, physical disability, or pain, while failing to address the societal ills that contribute to personal disease.[6] The recognition that the response to AIDS has been fueled by fear that borders on hysteria indicates that the church should be in the forefront of efforts to address pastorally both individual and societal concerns. This may require the church to speak both in pastoral terms and in prophetic concern to the issues surrounding the AIDS epidemic. The point has already been made that accepting a person with AIDS or ARC is not a matter of approving or disapproving a life-style, but of modeling for the community the church's unreserved love for one for whom Christ died. Paul reminds the Corinthians that they were *enlisted* in this ministry. His image is that of a people who are *conscripted*.

The church's pastoral care of AIDS or ARC patients, their loved ones, and their care-givers cannot be limited to personal acts of ministry or counseling. Pastoral ministry must include addressing the pervasive attitudes in society that isolate subgroups of citizens into categories of people who can then be dismissed—or rejected—in toto. And as surely as the church should address pastoral needs of oppressed groups, it also has an obligation to minister to the pastoral needs of a whole community. Society at large is afraid of AIDS and its consequences, and with good reason. The church must learn how to provide pastoral care both to those in need and to the community that is home to all. This latter pastoral role probably cannot be filled by individual clergy or church members, but represents a national function that requires compassionate leadership from the leaders of all religious communities, who, if they speak with one voice, can give expression to the church's pastoral care *of the nation*.

Third, the pastoral response to people affected by AIDS will be primarily a response to grief. One element appears to be characteristic of every affected person's life, the experience of loss that underlies every grief experience. Pastoral care of grieving patients, their parents and siblings, lovers, and care-givers becomes the context within which other aspects of ministry are set, including addressing questions of faith. The experience of loss overshadows every aspect of life. It actually comprises, to paraphrase Shakespeare's *Hamlet*, "battalions of losses." Unless this is recognized and addressed, other attempts at ministry may, at best, be merely ineffective and, at worst, will trivialize the effort to speak pastorally. Patients' losses include self-image and self-esteem, family relationships, home, friends, independence, physical mobility, the ability to perform simple tasks related to personal hygiene and preparing meals, and the devastating health losses: eyesight, mental acuity, speech, and continence. The threat of ultimate loss—death—is ever present.

Pastoral ministry will be effective only if the recognition of these losses is accompanied by a sensitive grief ministry that takes account of the shock and numbness, the anger and rage, and the depression that accompany loss. It is well known that a dying person's grief is paralleled by the grief of his or her entire circle of family and friends who are drawn into the vortex of loss. A sensitive ministry ought not be restricted to the "identified patient." Each person in the circle needs that ministry—including those care-givers who have become part of the dying person's "family," a phenomenon that frequently is present in the care of people with AIDS. Pastors should be reminded that it may be tempting at such moments to respond with what has been termed "self-serving or religiously imperialistic motives," resulting in misguided efforts to "save" people.[7] Such temptations should be resisted. To submit to them suggests that it is our individual efforts that rescue people, rather than that task being one that is within the reach only of the Holy Spirit.

Fourth, anger plays a role in the grief process. This is especially important to remember when caring for people with AIDS. It should not be surprising that people experiencing such catastrophic losses also will feel anger, even rage, toward their various situations. If one is angry with one's "situation," that anger is likely to be directed to the people who are nearest, including loved ones. People with AIDS or ARC are angry at their disease and the virus responsible for it. A few, but not many, are angry with God. What anger they have is displaced onto what might be perceived as relatively minor frustrations, but to which great importance is attached by the patient. For example, one patient made a phone inquiry to gain information from a governmental agency. His call was placed on hold, and he became increasingly frustrated as the wait was prolonged. Infuriated, he flung the phone away. He did not have time to waste sitting idly while a clerk took her time! This action may seem adolescent to a dispassionate observer, but to a dying person, time is not something he or she has to waste—there is so little time left.

In many situations intense levels of anger seem justified. For example, another patient's family became infuriated by the self-serving actions of the patient's immediate supervisor and the demeaning attitude expressed by excluding the patient from the company's building. Another parent stated: "My son has suffered enough from people from whom I expected at least some understanding and compassion. It is that type of failure that leaves me angry and in despair." Similar anger, often expressed in terms of frustration and despair, may be expressed by lovers and care-givers. It is important to understand that, while much of this anger is appropriate, it is also likely to express the helplessness and the anger derived from it that is evoked by the looming death of a patient one has grown to love. Being aware of these matters should help the pastor to minister with the deepest tenderness to the patient, family members, lover and hospital staff members.

Fifth, the pastor—ordained or lay minister—must count the cost of ministry. Pastoral presence entails both the time to be with people, unhurried by other concerns, and the readiness to enter the other person's world of pain—to the extent that it is ever possible for one person to enter another's world. Those who minister to people affected by AIDS need to have their own support system in place. The caring person inevitably will grieve as his or her life is touched by the pain and losses of others. In communities where patient or parental support groups are established, it is important for the sponsoring organization to provide opportunity for pastoral care of the staff members involved. If lay people are drawn into this ministry, it is incumbent on clergy to provide both supervision and support services. Clergy in whose congregation a member with AIDS has died have a particular opportunity to model acceptance of the family and friends through sensitive pastoral ministry, while ministering to the pastoral needs of the congregation qua congregation.

Pastoral care of the congregation may be facilitated by a pulpit ministry that offers a reasonable, informed, understanding presence and voice in addressing fears and prejudices and calling on the congregation to show acceptance and love. Themes that pastors may want to address include the redemptive impact of loving care, humility, and reconciliation. The pulpit ministry may be strengthened by a broader teaching ministry that is directed to a number of goals, for example, provision of accurate medical information, identification of the factors that are allowed—or used—to disrupt human relationships, and issues of life, death, and dying that are too easily evaded in a community that has tacitly denied the reality of death.

Specific ministries may be offered by the congregation to AIDS patients. These may include sacramental ministries; pastoral visits in person and by telephone; transportation to hospital or clinic; provision of meals, food pantry, shopping, housekeeping; housing and utility subsidies; sitting and basic nursing care; efforts at reconciliation; and support as a patient dies. Ministries to families and lovers may include emotional and spiritual support; respite from the stress of providing primary care; housing for out-of-town families; assistance in transportation (e.g., airports, hospitals); and support as a patient dies and during the period of grief. Care of the medical and institutional support staff—nurses, social workers, and physicians—is often overlooked but may be vital to the ability of a community to maintain adequate services. This ministry may include speaking to hospital staff members during visits to patients; pastoral care and counseling of staff members; and addressing theological meanings of illness and death.

These comments concerning pastoral care and proposals for specific congregational ministries are suggestive of the needs and opportunities for ministry occasioned by AIDS. Because the disease is unpredictable and the situations and needs of particular patients are variable, pastors and congregations may need to be creative in adapting their ministries to meet the specific needs and opportunities open to them.

STORIES NOT TOLD

The stories contained in this book are representative of the suffering and satisfaction experienced by people touched by AIDS. Every person's encounter with AIDS is unique. This book is not intended to provide a comprehensive description or analysis of the crisis of AIDS. But these stories are indicative of the defeats, victories, events, and emotions associated with this new disease. This type of introduction to the medical facts about AIDS, what it can do to people, and the church's responsibility with respect to it is a first step in overcoming the fears, identified in chapter 1, believed partially to explain the social and ecclesiastical response to AIDS.

People with AIDS or ARC, their families and lovers, and their health care providers have told their stories. The stories of other relevant people have not been told. They ought to be told because by doing so the full impact of AIDS could be better understood. For example, the stories of families who abandon a relative with AIDS or ARC deserve to be told. These people have been seen here indirectly. Every parent of this description whom the authors approached refused to participate in this project. Explanations were not given, only polite or impolite refusals. Other parents who journeyed with a son or daughter until death refused to share their experience with an anonymous audience. One mother said, "My son suffered with cancer for fifteen years before he died. Talking about it won't help him or me now." In fact, her son told her fifteen years ago that he was gay. He was diagnosed with Kaposi's sarcoma only fourteen months before he died. The embarrassment, anger, hurt, and grief implicit to both types of refusal suggest that the destruction and suffering caused by AIDS have only begun to be told by the narratives presented here.

A second category of stories is missing. These are the stories of families who know that a member is in a high-risk group for AIDS. Their fears and concerns, if known, would help to complete the picture of distress caused by AIDS. In addition, the stories of families who don't know but suspect that a member is in a high-risk group for AIDS are missing. Their fears and concerns probably take two forms, one having to do with the family member's risk factor (gay, bisexual, drug abuser) and the second having to do with the disease itself. Each type of family or situation adds another feature to the phenomenon of AIDS.

A third category of story not told, except indirectly, is the public's attitude toward and perception of AIDS and people with AIDS or ARC. Perhaps this information can be gathered from news reports, governmental action or inaction, and other institutional or individual responses (e.g., charities, social service agencies, professional associations, and religious denominations). The panic, on the one hand, and apathy, on the other hand, with which the public has responded to AIDS suggest that this public health problem has been politicized into a gay issue. A leading mayoral candidate in Houston stated that his solution to AIDS was to "shoot the queers." The candidate's campaign managers subsequently reported receiving a record amount of financial contributions the day after he made this remark. This incident and the reactions of some parents of children in school indicate that the public's story is complex and of crucial importance to understanding the full significance of AIDS.[8]

A fourth category of story not included here is that of the "worried-well" members of at-risk populations, especially gay and bisexual men. The anxiety and stress experienced by these people can be overwhelming. They grieve the loss of friends and worry if they will be next. They may forego relationships out of fear that the prospective partner may be contagious. They may refuse intimacies with others out of a concern not to risk infecting someone else. They may become overly concerned about their own health, becoming unreasonably alarmed about any sign or symptom of illness. But perhaps equally important, they may lose the will or ability to trust the people who have provided sanctuary in a hostile environment—other gay men.

The stories not told in this book and those that have been told indicate the extent of suffering caused by AIDS and ARC. The opportunities for ministry by pastors and congregations are significant. People who have been involved in this crisis since it began are rapidly being overwhelmed by the diverse needs associated with a growing population of patients. As important as participating in this service is, it is secondary to a more basic consideration—the identity and mission of the church. The church's response to AIDS will reflect how it sees itself in relation to the teaching and example of its Lord. The "poor," "dispossessed," and "outcast" for whom the prophets and Jesus had a special concern appear today as people with AIDS or ARC and, to a lesser degree, their loved ones and friends. For the church to ignore them and the varied needs that surround AIDS, to fail to respond in a redemptive manner, and to abandon a people who have almost no one to cry out in their behalf for mercy and justice would constitute an abdication of its mission and a corruption of its identity. The church is challenged by AIDS to be the church. May it have the will, commitment, and courage to meet the challenge. By so doing, it will not only follow Jesus' example, but also set an example for others to follow.

Notes _____

Chapter 1. AIDS and the Church

1. "AIDS," *Newsweek*, August 12, 1985, p. 20.
2. "Indiana School Told to Readmit 14-Year-Old Student with AIDS," *New York Times*, February 14, 1986, p. 8.
3. "Poll Finds Many AIDS Fears That the Experts Say Are Groundless," *New York Times*, September 12, 1985, p. 9.
4. For an interesting discussion of life plans, mortality, and risk budgets, see Charles Fried, *An Anatomy of Values* (Cambridge, MA: Harvard University Press, 1970), pp. 155–82.
5. Ernest Becker, *The Denial of Death* (New York: Free Press, 1973).
6. William Shakespeare, *Hamlet*, III, i, 79–82.
7. For a provocative reconceptualization of sexual morality and understandings from a Christian point of view, see James B. Nelson, *Embodiment* (Minneapolis: Augsburg Publishing House and New York: The Pilgrim Press, 1978). Two collections of philosophical analyses of sexual concepts and moral norms applied to sexual behavior are relevant to this discussion. Cf. Robert Baker and Frederick Elliston, eds., *Philosophy and Sex*, rev. ed. (Buffalo: Prometheus Books, 1984); and Alan Soble, ed., *Philosophy of Sex* (Totowa, NJ: Littlefield, Adams & Co., 1980).
8. Ronald Bayer, *Homosexuality and American Psychiatry* (New York: Basic Books, 1981).
9. George Weinberg's original discussion of homophobia continues to be instructive. See George Weinberg, *Society and the Healthy Homosexual* (Garden City, NY: Anchor Books, 1973).
10. Cited by Herb Hollinger, "Comments on Homosexuality Spur Removal," *Baptist Standard*, February 26, 1986, p. 11.
11. William E. Swing, " 'AIDS': How Should the Church Respond?" *The Living Church*, April 28, 1985, p. 8.

12. John R. Quinn, "The Archbishop's Response," *San Francisco Catholic,* September 1985, p. 9.

13. "Help for AIDS Victims," *The Christian Century,* February 26, 1986, pp. 201–2.

14. E.J. Hamlin, "Foreigner," *Interpreters Dictionary of the Bible,* vol. 2 (Nashville: Abingdon Press, 1962), 310–11.

15. Thomas W. Ogletree, *Hospitality to Strangers* (Philadelphia: Fortress Press, 1985), pp. 2–3, 7.

16. Earl E. Shelp and Ronald H. Sunderland, "AIDS and the Church," *The Christian Century,* September 11–18, 1985, pp. 797–800.

Chapter 2. Medical Facts About AIDS

1. Centers for Disease Control Task Force on Kaposi's Sarcoma and Opportunistic Infection, "Epidemiological Aspects of the Current Outbreak of Kaposi's Sarcoma and Opportunistic Infection," *New England Journal of Medicine* 306 (1982): 248–52.

2. J.L. Ziegler, A.C. Templeton, and C.L. Vogel, "Kaposi's Sarcoma: A Comparison of Classical Endemic and Endemic Forms," *Oncology* 11 (1984): 47–52.

3. J.M. Reuben et al., "Immunological Characterization of Homosexual Males," *Cancer Research* 43 (1983): 897–904, and E.M. Hersh et al., "Immunological Characterizations of Patients with AIDS, the AIDS-Related Symptom Complex and an AIDS-Related Life Style," *Cancer Research* 44 (1980): 5894–901.

4. V. Fainstein et al., "Disseminated Infection Due to Mycobacterium Avium Intercellular in a Homosexual Man with Kaposi's Sarcoma," *Journal of Infectious Diseases* 145 (1982): 586; S.D. Ditlik et al., "Cryptosporidial Cholecystitis," *New England Journal of Medicine* 308 (1983): 967; I. Garcia et al., "Nonbacterial Thrombotic Endocarditis in a Male Homosexual with Kaposi's Sarcoma," *Archives of Internal Medicine* 143 (1983): 1243–44; S.C. Pitlik et al., "Polymicrobial Brain Abcess in a Male Homosexual with Kaposi's Sarcoma," *Southern Medical Journal* 77 (1984): 271–72; S.H. Stein et al., "Celiac Disease and Cytomegalovirus Esophagitis in a Homosexual Man with Acquired Immune Deficiency: A Case Report," unpublished manuscript.

5. J.L. Ziegler et al., "Non-Hodgkin's Lymphoma in Homosexual Men with Lymphadenopathy or AIDS: Clinical Features in 90 Patients from Six Institutions," *New England Journal of Medicine* 311 (1984): 565–70.

6. G.R. Newell et al., "Risk Factor Analysis Among Men Referred for Possible AIDS," *Preventive Medicine,* in press; and E.M. Hersh et al., "Effects of the Recreational Agent Isobutyl Nitrite on Human

Peripheral Blood Leukocytes: Evidence for a Non-specific Cytotoxic Effect," *Cancer Research* 43 (1983): 1365–71.

7. G.M. Mavligit et al., "Chronic, Sperm-Induced Allo-Antigenic Stimulation: A New Hypothesis for Immune Dysregulation in Homosexual Males," *Journal of the American Medical Association* 251 (1984): 237–41.

8. J.W. Curran, "The Epidemiology and Prevention of the Acquired Immunodeficiency Syndrome," *Annals of Internal Medicine* 103 (1985): 657–62.

9. L. Montagnier et al., "Adaptation of Lymphadenopathy Associated Virus (LAV) to Replication in EBV-Transformed B Lymphoblastoid Cell Lines," *Science* 225 (1984): 63–66.

10. R.C. Gallo et al., "Frequent Detection and Isolation of Cytopathic Retroviruses (HTLV-III) from patients with AIDS and At Risk for AIDS," *Science* 224 (1984): 500–503.

11. J.A. Levy, "Isolation of Lymphocytopathic Retroviruses from San Francisco Patients with AIDS," *Science* (1984): 840–42.

12. W.D. Snider et al., "Neurological Complications of Acquired Immune Deficiency Syndrome Analysis of 50 Patients," *Annals of Neurology* 14 (1983): 403–18, and S.D. Pitlik et al., "Spectrum of Central Nervous System Complications in Male Homosexuals with Acquired Immuno-deficiency Syndrome," *Journal of Infectious Diseases* 148 (1983): 771–72.

13. R. Edelman and J. Kellen, "AIDS-Related Complex: A Definition," *AIDS Memorandum* 1 (1984): 1–16.

14. T.J. Spira et al., "Prevalence of Antibody to Lymphadenopathy—Associated Virus Among Drug-Detoxification Patients in New York, *New England Journal of Medicine* 311 (1984): 467–68, and J. Laurence et al., "Lymphadenopathy Associated Viral Antibody in AIDS Immune Correlations and Definitions of Carrier State," *New England Journal of Medicine* 311 (1984): 1269–73.

15. John Langone, "AIDS," *Discover,* December 1985, p. 28.

16. J.B. Brunet and R.A. Ancelle, "The International Occurrence of the Acquired Immune Deficiency Syndrome," *Annals of Internal Medicine* 103 (1985): 670–74, and P. Piot et al., "Acquired Immunodeficiency Syndrome in a Heterosexual Population in Zaire," *Lancet* 2 (1984): 377–79.

17. G.N. Holland et al., "Acquired Immune Deficiency Syndrome Ocular Manifestations," *Ophthalmology* 90 (1983): 859–73, and P.R. Rosenberg et al., "Acquired Immunodeficiency Syndrome Ophthalmic Manifestations in Ambulatory Patients," *Ophthalmology* 90 (1983): 874–78.

18. A.M. Hardy et al., "The Economic Impact of the First 10,000 Cases of Acquired Immunodeficiency Syndrome in the United States," *Journal of the American Medical Association* 255 (1986): 209–11.

Chapter 4. Families and Lovers

1. Larry Henley and Jeff Silbar, "Wind Beneath My Wings" (Bobby Goldsboro Music, Inc. and House of Gold Music, Inc., 1982).

Chapter 6. Pastoral Perspectives and Recommendations

1. Cf. Earl E. Shelp and Ronald H. Sunderland, eds., *The Pastor as Servant* (New York: The Pilgrim Press, 1986).

2. Cf. Earl E. Shelp and Ronald H. Sunderland, eds., *The Pastor as Prophet* (New York: The Pilgrim Press, 1985).

3. Eric Cassell has thoughtfully written from a physician's perspective on the subject of healing in terms other than curing. See Eric J. Cassell, *The Healer's Art* (Cambridge, MA: MIT Press, 1985).

4. Numerous studies have appeared recently that challenge the claims that homosexual people are condemned by God and that homosexual conduct is sin. See George R. Edwards, *Gay/Lesbian Liberation* (New York: The Pilgrim Press, 1984), John Boswell, *Christianity, Social Tolerance, and Homosexuality* (Chicago: University of Chicago Press, 1980), James B. Nelson, *Embodiment* (Minneapolis: Augsburg Publishing House and New York: The Pilgrim Press, 1978), Letha Scanzoni and Virginia Ramey Mollenkott, *Is the Homosexual My Neighbor?* (San Francisco: Harper & Row, 1978), and W. Norman Pittenger, *Making Sexuality Human* (New York: The Pilgrim Press, 1970).

5. For a complete discussion of the metaphor of "sustaining presence" applied to persons in the helping professions, see Earl E. Shelp, "Courage: A Neglected Virtue in the Patient-Physician Relationship," *Social Science and Medicine*, November 1983, pp. 417–29; see also Earl E. Shelp, *Born to Die?* (New York: Free Press, 1986), pp. 92–98.

6. One of the first people to address this issue was Donald Browning. His article "Pastoral Care and Public Ministry," *The Christian Century*, September 28, 1966, pp. 175–77, provides a concise discussion of the need to integrate public and pastoral ministry.

7. Cf. James A. Wharton, "Theology and Ministry in the Hebrew Scriptures," *A Biblical Basis for Ministry*, Earl E. Shelp and Ronald Sunderland, eds. (Philadelphia: Westminster Press, 1981), pp. 49–53. Wharton warns pastoral carers against the temptation to perceive their work as directed toward "saving" people. He adds: "I may sail into the task [of ministry to another] with the exalted notion that it is my job to intervene in the lives of others, and to secure for them a

kind of well-being that only I can provide. But it is at just such points that the biblical word says to us: 'Don't take yourself so seriously!' Neither our well-being nor the well-being of the other rests ultimately in our own hands. It is a liberating gift of God" (p. 69).

8. Cf. Dennis Altman, *AIDS in the Mind of America* (Garden City, NY: Anchor Press, 1986).